WRONG HORSE

WRONG ROOMS

Also by Mark Sanderson

FICTION
Audacious Perversion

NON-FICTION
The Making of Inspector Morse
Don't Look Now (BFI Modern Classic)

WRONG ROOMS

A Memoir

Mark Sanderson

Scribner

First published in Great Britain by Scribner in 2002
An imprint of Simon & Schuster UK Ltd
A Viacom company

3 5 7 9 10 8 6 4 2

Simon & Schuster UK Ltd
Africa House
64–78 Kingsway
London WC2B 6AH

Simon & Schuster Australia
Sydney

www.simonsays.co.uk

A CIP catalogue for this book is available
from the British Library.

ISBN: 0-7432-2009-9

Typeset in Baskerville MT by M Rules
Printed and bound in Great Britain by
Mackays of Chatham plc, Chatham, Kent

To our parents

CONTENTS

CONTENTS

'It was the nature of his profession that his experience with death should be greater than most and he said that while it was true that time heals bereavement it does so only at the cost of the slow extinction of those loved ones from the heart's memory which is the sole place of their abode then or now. Faces fade, voices dim. Seize them whispered the *sepulturero*. Speak with them. Call their names. Do this and do not let sorrow die for it is the sweetening of every gift . . .'

—CORMAC MCCARTHY, *The Crossing*

AUTHOR'S NOTE

I have called this book *Wrong Rooms* because Drew and I both saw places we never expected to see. The blinkers were ripped from our eyes. We entered a grave new world of waiting rooms, consulting rooms, hospital wards and theatres. The fact that our lives had only just changed for the better made the shock even worse.

Drew made me happier than I had ever been before. He took me to places I never expected to see. His death left me bereft and, stupid with grief, I found myself in more wrong rooms and, eventually, took the wrong way out. What follows is both a celebration and a confession.

I have pieced together the evidence from diaries, notes, letters and videos. Our friends and families have provided me with additional testimony. None of them knew the whole truth until now. Most of the material was already in my head:

the memory can be an amazing – and frightening – thing. Some names have been changed to protect the guilty.

My life with Drew has seemed more real to me than any subsequent period. It was as if the clock had stopped on 16 July 1994. Writing *Wrong Rooms* has started the clock ticking again, even if it does occasionally strike thirteen. It was the only way I could bring Drew back to life. However, he could not speak for himself so there are times when I have had to put words into his mouth. This was easy enough: I still talk to him every day.

PROLOGUE

The fresh whitewash dazzled in the afternoon sun. I placed the two red roses – one from my mother, one from myself – on Drew's grave. Ants – twice the size of any in Britain – swarmed over the painted concrete. I brushed them off and perched on a corner of the tomb. 'Hello, Possum. I'm back.'

Eighteen months had passed since my last visit and yet a part of me, the best part of me, had never left this place. I often returned to it in my mind's eye. The wattle tree and the allamanda had vanished. They must have died. One day my remains would end up here too. A Qantas jet, banking overhead, drowned out the exotic birdsong.

I did not cry until I left the cemetery: walking away was always the hardest part.

*

I was in Cairns to talk to Drew's parents. I had now known them three times as long as I had known their son. Their home was only a few minutes away. However, I was not yet ready. I was facing the most difficult conversation of my life. After seven years another couple of hours would make no difference.

I crossed the Captain Cook Highway by the Tobruk Swimming Pool and made my way over the vast playing fields to the Esplanade. A shaggy-haired man in a pair of Day-Glo orange shorts dive-bombed a clump of palm trees with his kite. In the distance a succession of ships brought their cargo of day-trippers back from the Reef. I would return to the hotel, have a shower, then telephone Jack and Aileen. If writing the book had been difficult, telling them the truth was going to be even harder.

The stones lining the drive — no doubt painted with the same whitewash as the grave — glowed in the taxi's headlights. Aileen stood silhouetted in the front door of the old Queenslander. Jasper, Drew's pet cockatoo, who lived under the house, screeched a welcome. I climbed the wooden steps as though mounting my own scaffold. I hugged Drew's mother. The animosity that I had first felt towards her had gradually turned into love. The long hot summer days of 1994 had been filled with pain. Now I was going to cause more grief. It was 5 November 2001. The next day was her birthday. I gave her the present I had bought at Heathrow. 'No peeping till tomorrow.'

Jack emerged from the kitchen. We shook hands. His grip was as firm as ever. On the last occasion I had seen him he was recovering from a heart operation. Now he was due to have an operation on his eyes. My timing could not have been worse. On the other hand, there was never going to be a good time to tell them what I had to say.

Aileen opened a bottle of sparkling wine. The television news jabbered on about the rapidly approaching General Election. Ming-Ming, an ancient Siamese, rubbed his bony body against my leg. I gave Jack a Roman coin that Drew had bought when he visited Hadrian's Wall. I did not want him to feel left out. He collected all sorts of things, especially shells. A few of his most prized specimens, including a giant conch, were displayed in a glass cabinet at the back of the room. Drew had shared his love of the sea.

It was hot and humid. Back in England, even in the depths of winter, Drew would pad around the flat in bare feet. He had spent more time on sand than carpet. His parents' home, the house he had grown up in, had polished wooden floors. He had sat where I was sitting. If only he could be here with me now.

The alcohol went straight to my head. I was sweating from fear as well as the heat but was grateful for the Dutch courage. The electric fans whirred. Our small talk burbled on. I looked at the photograph of Drew on the wall. I had taken it myself on our first – and last – holiday. 'Just do it,' said the voice. 'Do it now!'

I drained my glass. I cleared my throat. The moment I had been dreading for months had finally arrived. I had kept silent for too long. Jack and Aileen had a right to know what had happened in that room in Packington Street. I should have told them sooner. My only consolation was that I had not left it too late.

'There's something that you need to know. You won't thank me for telling you but it's important that you hear it from me.' His mother and father looked up. I had travelled halfway round the world to reach this point. Their reaction would affect the rest of my life.

'When Drew knew he was going to die I made him a promise. I never expected to have to keep it but . . . I did. I kept my promise.'

LONELY HEARTS

Your life can change at any moment, whether you want it to or not. Sometimes it is easy to recognise the moment – passing an examination, proposing marriage, finding your lover in bed with someone else – but the most radical shift often occurs without you even realising it at the time. Oncoming trucks are easier to spot than soulmates.

It was the summer of 1992. French lorry-drivers were blockading holiday routes throughout France. French and British trawlers were ramming each other off the Isles of Scilly. However, deep in the Gers, in the south-west of the country, the only breach of the peace was birdsong. I was staying with friends in a converted barn near Fleurance. Our long, lazy lunch was over. We were lolling on the banks of the lake that gave the house its name. A gentle breeze shimmered across the surface of the water. Even in the shade of the poplars, it was hot.

Nick, whose sister owned Le Lac, was reading *Under God* by Garry Wills in a deck-chair. The Tweety-Pie baseball cap on his head did not suit him but the television executive was making a statement: 'I am on holiday.' Jo, his wife, one of my former colleagues from *Time Out* magazine, was playing with Isabelle, their three-year-old daughter. Janine, their shy Australian nanny, lay in the sun listening to her Walkman. I was doing nothing – and finding it very difficult. Holidays always seemed more fun in anticipation or in hindsight. Relaxing was hard work.

There was a distant crunch of tyres on gravel. Everyone looked up. A car turned off the road and bounced its way up the long drive to the house. Cerby, short for Cerberus, started barking. The Great Dane was friendlier than his name suggested and seemed to understand English as well as French. Doors slammed. The housekeeper emerged and pointed to the lake. Nick and Jo waved to the new arrivals. The couple waved back and started strolling hand-in-hand down the hill towards us. Cerby padded back to his post on the terrace.

Pascal and Marta were celebrating their first wedding anniversary. He worked in television; she in journalism. When the introductions were over Jo, Isabelle and Janine took Marta back to the house so she could unpack. Pascal continued chatting with Nick for ten minutes and then said he fancied a swim. He apologised for not having any trunks and stripped off. He stretched his perfect limbs in the sun, slowly, and waded into the lake. The water was ice-cold but he did not make a sound.

I was not sure which I admired most: his nonchalance or his physique. I suddenly saw myself through his eyes: just one more pallid, lonely Englishman out of condition and out of his depth. I put my T-shirt back on and went up to the house.

My thirtieth birthday was looming and yet I was as single and frustrated as I had been at seventeen. I still had no real idea of who I was, what I was doing or where I was going. One thing was certain, though: things had to change.

On Halloween, 1991, I hailed a cab at the Aldwych in the heart of London. It had been a typical day. I had spent the morning at Channel 4 watching television documentaries on persecution in Spain; concentration camps in Czechoslovakia; fossils in India; hospitals in Ghana; and film-making in Vietnam – plus a celebration of flautist James Galway's fiftieth birthday – and spent the afternoon writing reviews of them at the *Time Out* office in Covent Garden. I had, as was usual, been out for lunch with colleagues in between – and, as was usual, drunk one and a half bottles of wine.

'You know, for a split second then, Mark, I saw what you'll look like when you're old.' Everyone had studied my incipient jowls with amusement. The fact that I did not see the joke had made them laugh all the more.

'Still at *Time Out* then?'

'Sorry?'

The cabbie winked in the rear-view mirror. 'I picked you up at the same place a while ago. Write about TV and stuff, don't you? We had a good chat. Life's treating you well, I see.'

Cities are not as anonymous as we like to think. Stuck in our ruts, following our daily routines, we are bound to collide with the same fellow wage-slaves occasionally. 'Stay in Piccadilly Circus long enough,' my father would say, 'and you'll eventually see everyone you know.' It was not an encouraging thought. I had come to the capital in search of freedom, not familiarity.

I left *Time Out* the following month. Freelance journalists could not afford to go out for lunch every day. I drank less and travelled more: to California with the cast and crew of *Byker Grove*, the long-running children's drama series, to file a location report for the *Radio Times*; and to Spain, for *The Times*, to explain how owning a bar on the Costa del Sol is by no means as much fun as many British holidaymakers imagine. I even finished writing my third novel.

I had been working hard, but not working out. I accepted Jo's invitation to France because I knew I needed a rest. However, the skinny-dipping Frenchman reminded me that I had not had sex for over a year. I was still recovering from a love affair that had ended badly. The self-proclaimed television presenter – who seemed to spend most of his time as a continuity announcer – had made my life a misery. Nicknamed 'TVP' by my friends, the only person he loved was himself. I still jumped when I occasionally heard his voice, introducing quiz programmes on Channel 4: a real-life ghost in the machine.

Pascal increased the pressure I felt to shape up mentally and physically. I had to get my confidence back. The answer lay literally around the corner.

That summer the disused laundry in Milton Grove, Stoke Newington, had been converted into a private gym. Many of my colleagues at *Time Out* used to go across the road to work out at Jubilee Hall at lunchtime, but I had preferred raising a wine-glass to lifting weights. Either way you returned to your desk red-faced and sweating. Besides, I did not want them to see me with no clothes on. That was why I had refused the invitations of friends – most of whom belonged to a gym – to join them for a work-out: the thought of being found wanting by a shower of muscle queens was enough to make anyone shrink in terror.

I stayed at home reading and writing. Alex, my best friend, dubbed me 'The Hermit of Shakespeare Walk', and in a sense he was right. I often came home on a Friday night, locked the door behind me, and did not re-emerge till Monday morning. Work, household chores, television and newspapers filled the days. Time would only begin to drag late on Sunday afternoon. The period between 5 and 6pm was the nadir of the week. It was when my parents had dropped me off at boarding school after a weekend exeat or holiday. Almost twenty years later my spirits still sank under the weight of remembered dread. I was afraid of remaining single yet tired of running after unsuitable partners. However, unless I took action now, a life of quiet desperation was the best I could expect. The fact that I was still alone at twenty-nine suggested there was something wrong with me. I had to at least try to remedy the situation.

Milton Grove backed on to Shakespeare Walk. It was not as if I were going out of my way. So, on a sunny afternoon in

August, I stepped through the doors of the N16 gym for the first time.

The walls of the vast weights room were lined with mysterious pieces of equipment. The floor-to-ceiling windows had been replaced with glass bricks. Good: passers-by could not stare in. The ranks of exercise bikes and rowing machines all stood idle. A single, reassuringly fat, man huffed and puffed on a stretch mat, his eyes glued to MTV. And that, apart from a deserted café and the changing rooms, was it. I made an appointment for a fitness test with a taciturn teenager called Jason. One minute later I was back in my flat.

I could not believe I had done it. I had hated games at school – I preferred the loneliness of the long-distance runner to the heartiness of team sports – and, after the fifth form, had taken no part in them. If only meaty, moody Mr Sutcliffe had said, 'Look, Mark, physical exercise develops your figure. The boys won't fancy you unless you have a slim waist, tight buns and big biceps' I would have been scrumming down with the rest of them, and maybe even enjoying it. I had not known what I liked in those days. Now I knew what I wanted.

Alex had been an early starter. He had even slept with one of his teachers. He had always led the life I wished to lead. Better-looking, and better-off, he was the man I might have been. He already had a boyfriend when I met him at the University of Manchester in 1982. I was reading English Language and Literature; he was doing American Studies. Even then I spent my time looking back, whereas Alex was usually one step ahead. His self-assurance and unabashed hedonism intrigued and intimidated me. He took one look at my wardrobe, made me fill out an application form for a credit card and was soon introducing me to the joys of recreational shopping. Anything was more fun than Anglo-Saxon.

Alex's specialist subject was men. He gave me a crash course in them. We became fixtures in The Stuffed Olive (owned by a man called Clive) and High Society, basement bars which crammed everyone into a single room and then deafened them with hi-NRG hits such as 'Earthquake' and 'Searching'. We were known as 'The Two Virgins': most disco bunnies did not know the meaning of discretion. One night we were persuaded to take part in a swimwear competition. Alex came second and I came nowhere – even though I had kept my T-shirt on. The fact that I even agreed to mince round the dance-floor half-naked now fills me with amazement. It was the early 1980s, though, and body fascism was still just a crazy cult in California.

If Alex got me into a lot of trouble – the bedrooms of married men, waiting rooms in doctors' surgeries, the bank manager's office – he also got me out of it. We shared a flat in our final year, next-door to the swimming baths in Hathersage Road, yet both of us managed to graduate with honours and a 2.1 degree.

'Who'd want to wake up next to you?' Alex helped himself to another chocolate digestive. 'You'll have to stop buying these if you really want to lose weight.'

I was accustomed to Alex's sharp tongue but his words

still stung. What was the point of going to a gym if you could not eat what you wanted? It was the hardest thing I had ever done. Each Monday, Wednesday and Friday morning I dragged myself to N16. I could not get Jason's pitying gaze, as he had fixed the heartbeat sensors to my naked, sagging chest, out of my head. The test had established that I was fit enough to exercise but a long way from being fit. I followed his regime of two sets of twelve repetitions on each of the Nautilus machines religiously. I pulled on the Concept II rowing machine until I nearly fainted. I ached all the time, I was hungry all the time, but my spare tyre had started to deflate. To begin with, ashamed of my puniness, I had increased the weight on a machine when I had finished using it, but now I no longer bothered. Fellow off-peak members had even started to say hello to me. I was drinking less because I found it impossible to train with a hangover. And I was slowly getting used to being in the company of naked men again. It was early days but, to be honest, I was secretly proud of myself.

Alex, however, was not impressed. His biceps had long been ten times the size of mine. He drank special powders to bulk up his muscles. I hit back at his gibe by telling him that I had met a boy called Sam. The sauna had suddenly got much hotter when, during an idle conversation about being a television reviewer, he had asked me if my name was Mark Sanderson. Sam had seen a copy of a book I had written about *Inspector Morse* when he had recently gone back to Alex's house for sex. Alex had picked him up on a street in Bloomsbury one lunchtime. So much for anonymity.

Sam was darkly handsome. My heart had melted when, straining on the overhead press, he had flashed me a rueful smile. It was typical of Alex that he had already been to bed with him. He always got what I wanted.

When I told Alex that I had decided to place an advertisement in *Time Out* he immediately decided to do the same. 'You write it for me. You're much better at these things than me. You've had a lot of practice.'

It was true. In those days, if you did not like shouting at strangers in smoky pubs and clubs, there was no other way of meeting gay men. I found it difficult to communicate without words. How could you show a sense of humour without them? Chat lines and chat rooms were years away. Trolling around Hampstead Heath was too dangerous: you never knew what was lurking in the bushes. The very idea of cottaging – sex in public lavatories – repelled me. However, a good Lonely Hearts ad could widen your circle of friends if nothing else.

It took me five minutes to write Alex's advert and five days to concoct my own. It was important to create an immediate impression, to catch the eye. You had to appear confident, serious and desirable, not cocky, frivolous and desperate. It would have been easier to compose a haiku. The three lines came to represent a last chance for romance.

In the event the two ads appeared together in the issue of *Time Out* for the week of 9–16 September 1992. Alex, as usual, led the way. He had chosen to pay extra for a semi-display ad: 'It's only right that I stand out.'

EVERYTHING BUT THE BOY
**Stunning athletic gay guy, 28, seeks intelligent
and very good-looking soul-mate (25–35) to
share his successful but single life.
Telephone and photo essential. Box 387**

---

* SUCCESSFUL WRITER, 29, gay, tall, dark, handsome,
seeks non-smoking, significant other 25–35, to share love
of cinema, good food, and maybe the Sunday papers.
Photo, telephone essential. Box 388

A week later we received our first replies. I walked round to
Alex's flat in Highbury. It was much bigger than my own
place, and in a more desirable area, but St Paul's Road was
still a comedown from the house he had until recently shared
with Robert, his lover of nine years. Their bruising break-up
had affected me deeply. I had watched their relationship grow
ever since we had all been at Manchester together: such intimacy and security represented my ideal of domesticity. I was
almost as fond of Robert as I was of Alex, and had warned my
best friend not to lose him. Rob was handsome, young and
rich. What more did he want? Alex, of course, knew better.
It was not working, so he walked. Affairs make people unhappy
because only unhappy people have them in the first place.

We compared and contrasted the contenders over pizza
and champagne. Alex had attracted ten and I had netted six.
Three people had replied to both of us and went straight into
the bin (they were not very good-looking anyway). I had

already been to bed with one of the others – a South African soldier who, at the vital moment, had exclaimed, 'Suffer like a Kaffir!' That left me with two: a stocky, blond cook and a skinny, ginger accountant.

On 25 September I walked to the Angel to buy *Monopolies of Loss* by Adam Mars-Jones. When I got back the postman had been. The big brown envelope contained eleven more replies. Seven correspondents were hopeless, three would be all right – if nothing better came along – and the last one had written a lecture on white air-mail paper:

13 September 1992

Mr Drew F. Morgan
23 Winifred St
Swindon
Wiltshire
SN3 1RT

Dear Mr Box 388,
     I feel slightly daunted writing what amounts to a personal letter to a perfect stranger, but as nobody's perfect I shall forge ahead.
     The first revelation I must needs make is that I am an Australian over here on a two-year working holiday visa (I arrived mid-February of this year). If you have the unfortunate habit of watching Australian soaps . . . well

there's probably a lot more to Australia than will be divined from the residents of Ramsay Street. A brief aside about Australia will not be out of place at this point: [There followed a hand-drawn map of Australia showing the state boundaries and the cities of Perth, Darwin, Cairns, Brisbane, Sydney, Canberra, Melbourne, Hobart and Adelaide.]

I grew up in Cairns, next to the Great Barrier Reef, but now live and work in Brisbane (the capital of the Sunshine State). I still have a job in Brisbane and was granted leave without pay to come over to England. Thanks to being in the Commonwealth and under 28 I was entitled to a two-year working holiday visa. I turn 28 in December of this year, but as I already have the visa it will run its extent. You may have heard of the very liberal laws regarding gays in New South Wales and Victoria – Sydney (the capital of NSW) is known worldwide for the Gay Mardi Gras that takes place each year. But Queensland, just north of NSW, until recently was held firmly in the iron grip of the National Party who were determined to cling to a false veneer of Victorian sexual mores. I say a false veneer for while persecuting gays, the government of Queensland was brought down by corruption charges for its involvement in crime, racketeering, prostitution, gambling . . . etc. Still, until late 1990, with a more open-minded Labour government at the helm, homosexuality was decriminalised. Sodomy and gay acts can still be punished with imprisonment, but slowly Queensland is being dragged screaming into the 1990s. Needless to say, growing up under such an oppressive anti-gay regime, and working for the government, has led me to become a very careful, straight-acting person. While Britain too is fighting for further gay legislation it is still a breath of freedom to me. You may wonder why I put up with Queensland and didn't simply move to NSW or Victoria. The answer relies on a knowledge of how beautiful Queensland is – politics aside. Sun-drenched, golden, sandy beaches, crashing waves, tropical rainforests, wide open spaces, glorious weather. People from the southern states may disagree, but if that were true, why do so many of them move to Queensland? We in Queensland say that the only good thing to come out of Victoria and NSW is the road to Queensland. Anyway, enough of such things, I merely mentioned them to give background to me.

By profession I am an analyst programmer who specialises in CSP, SQL, DB2 and Cobol on IBM mainframes. I contract my services to companies. At present I have a contract with a firm in Swindon, hence the reason why I live here. Although Swindon is an abominable place, it is surrounded by beautiful, even enchanting countryside – Iron Age forts, stone circles and the oldest Iron Age road in Europe. I explored all these facets on long walks with rangers from the local parks. Swindon is also very central to Oxford, Bath, Salisbury and even Stratford-upon-Avon. That said, now I've been here 4 months, it is probably time to move on somewhere else and commute to work. I have managed so far to avoid purchasing a car but may soon need to do so if I choose to live in Oxford. There's even a possibility that I may return to London and catch a train out daily. We shall see. Wherever I am I will not be averse to travelling. Distances mean different things to Australians as opposed to British people. If the reasons (or person) were right I would willingly travel considerable lengths. After all, most of my family still live in Cairns and I didn't blink to consider popping 2,000km north of Brisbane to visit them.

So, I've told you I program computers . . . merely one arrow to my bow. I actually gave up computers several years ago and did a one-year Graduate Diploma in Teaching Primary. I really wanted to teach primary school children, but due to my Bachelor of Science and the desperate need for maths/science teachers, I was placed in a high school. I taught for almost a year and was teaching the equivalent of your A and O-levels (the last time I'd seen some of the material was when I was at school!). It is a crying shame, but little wonder those emerging from school are only partially educated. They refused to transfer me to primary school so I resigned and returned to computers. In the years since I have completed a Bachelor of Arts with a major in each of English Literature and Ancient History. The degree was undertaken part-time of course, as I was working during the day. I have written a few short stories – science fiction and fantasy mostly – but after studying Ancient Rome, with its political intrigue, sexual decadence and the interplay of events that shaped the future of Europe, I have now started researching what I hope will be my first novel. I must confess to having done nothing towards it while over here as I have been rather preoccupied, but I'm in no hurry. I still have more research to complete before putting pen to paper on a dramatisation of the brothers Gracchi.

My list of interests also includes: reading, tennis (badly), badminton, board games, Role Master (a variation on Dungeons and Dragons), aerobics, going to the beach, listening to music (rock, pop, classical, opera), going to the theatre and cinema, staying in to watch TV and videos, sometimes cooking, and going for lots of long walks. Considering this list, there are two aspects about me which may strike you as incongruous: I cannot swim and I do not have a tan (by Australian standards). I just love the beach though and am content to paddle in the shallow breakers, build sandcastles or just lie enveloped in 15+ sunscreen. You may not have cause to worry in Britain, yet, but in Australia skin cancer is very serious – and a killer. So I don't expose myself unnecessarily; but I still like the beach and this is perhaps what I miss most about Queensland.

My personal particulars are: 5ft 7½ins, dark brown hair tending to bronze in some places, clear blue eyes (my best feature so many people tell me), fair skin (by Australian standards), slim, non-smoking, clean-living, honest, reliable, I attend church with a sort of regularity (though I have a very open mind regarding religious beliefs – so please do not be put off by this fact) and lastly, though definitely not least, I have a really bad sense of humour, being notorious among my friends for telling really pathetic jokes.

By now you are turned on, turned off, interested to find out more or something else. I can sometimes come across as pompous in letters (but I'm trying to change this) and certainly do not intend to sound as though I'm blowing my own trumpet. But what else do you say in a letter of this nature? The ball is, of course, definitely now in your court. There is no telephone where I am presently staying but my work number is (0793) 616161 extension 2356. You will naturally be ultra-discreet. I look forward to your response.

Yours faithfully
DREW F. MORGAN

PS: Do not take the photo too seriously – I am not overly photogenic.

Great. Just what I needed: a sci-fi-loving computer nerd who told lousy jokes. However, his letter stood out for several reasons. It was very long – twenty times as long as all the other replies put together – and very serious. It must have taken ages to write – and by hand too. It made all the other photocopied scrawls and scribbled notes seem like the cynical bids for easy sex they were. Then again, a stranger in a strange land, he probably had plenty of time on his hands: Swindon was not known for its nightlife. But what was the point of getting to know someone who would be back on the other side of the world in less than eighteen months?

I looked at the photograph again. It had been taken in a cemetery. Drew seemed cute enough. For some reason he was squatting between two old gravestones. There was something written on the back: 'This is one of my favourite pictures. I don't know why, I just like it. Now it is yours.'

I picked up the phone – and changed our lives.

2

FIREWORKS

I did not get through to Drew straight away. He was in a meeting so I left an 'ultra-discreet' message. Ninety minutes later he called back. We had a brief chat but I could tell he was inhibited by his surroundings. I liked the sound of his voice. There was nothing harsh about his Australian twang. He said he was always being mistaken for a South African or a Kiwi: 'We all sound the same to you Brits.'

As agreed, I sent Drew a photograph. It showed me on the prow of a San Francisco ferry: pink-faced from the Californian sun of the day before rather than embarrassment at being watched by a mob of unsmiling early-morning commuters. The *Byker Grove* film crew had made all the sarcastic remarks necessary. I wrote my telephone number on the back: 'If this has not put you off, call me!' Two days later he did.

Thereafter we spoke on the phone every day. Sometimes

for a couple of hours, sometimes for just a few minutes. We may have paused for breath occasionally but an awkward silence never occurred. Although we came from opposite sides of the globe, there seemed to be some common ground between us. Both our fathers were dentists, and his father and I shared a birthday: 16 November. Pure coincidence, of course, but it felt as though we were fated to meet.

We did so at the Barbican. The arts centre is built on the site of a watch-tower, part of the ancient fortifications designed to protect the City of London. The area was heavily bombed during the Blitz. I did not know it at the time, but I too would soon be under siege.

After years of similar meetings, hastily arranged dates that led only to brief encounters, I could not help judging by appearance. When I saw the short, smart young man marching towards me my immediate reaction was 'No'. I have never been more wrong. We shook hands. Drew was not as good-looking as I had expected. That was the trouble with telephone romances: the idealised picture you formed of your potential partner was bound to suffer in comparison with the real thing. We strolled, slightly embarrassed by the artificiality of the arrangement, into the waterside café. I grabbed a sandwich and waited for Drew to decide what he wanted. He took ages. What was the matter with him? My butterflies gave way to curiosity.

We spent the afternoon in The Pit watching a performance of Billy Roche's play, *Amphibians*. We both responded to the dilemmas faced by the characters, caught as they are between childhood and maturity, land and sea, their desire to belong at

odds with an urge to escape. It was getting dark when we surfaced. We could have gone our separate ways then and there,
yet the thought did not cross my mind. I already liked being
with him. Besides, neither of us had anything better to do. It
was Saturday night. We wandered round Soho and had tea in
a café in Beak Street.

Drew seemed quite uptight at first. I attributed this to
nerves: he had been less reticent on the telephone. Forced to
make conversation, I fell into my usual role as an interviewer,
asking questions and trying to decide whether or not the
answers were truthful. I soon learned that Drew never lied. If
his shyness had nothing to do with nerves, was he simply
having second thoughts? I knew, on first acquaintance, I could
be too much for some people: too overpowering, too up-
front, too in-your-face. I did take a little getting used to.
There was only one way to find out. 'Like to come back to my
place?'

We watched a James Bond movie, *The Living Daylights*, on
television and shared a bottle of champagne. Drew was not
too keen on the taste. He confessed that if he drank alcohol at
all he preferred a sweeter wine, such as Mateus Rosé. Mateus
Rosé? He had to be kidding. No one actually drank such
muck. Cheap Italian restaurants simply used the empty bottles as candlesticks. No wonder the Bollinger seemed rather
dry. Still, it did the trick. The boy from Oz relaxed into my
arms. We went to bed.

We stayed there until lunchtime the following day. We
waded through the papers together – fulfilling one part of the
ad at least – and had sex once again, just like couples were

supposed to do on a Sunday morning. He freaked out when I said, playing with the crucifix round his neck, 'You realise you'll burn in hell after this.' I was only teasing. He explained that the chain was unusually long because he did not wish to make a show of his religion: 'You can't see the cross even if my collar's open. My parents gave it to me on my twenty-first birthday.' I fell into a fitful doze. It had not been a good night. Drew snored. He blamed the champagne.

We bathed together, Drew continuing to soak while I made brunch. He emerged from the bathroom holding his towel rather than wrapping it round his waist. My eyes followed him into the bedroom. He had a good body, compact, chunky, not at all tanned. His bottom, surprisingly muscular, was his best feature, and he made sure I saw it.

After we had eaten, Drew watched a tape of *Blade Runner*, one of his favourite films, while I compiled a photo-montage of me, my family and friends to hang in the kitchen. It provided Drew with a crash-course in my recent history. He seemed genuinely interested. Then again, he was astonishingly polite. When he left to catch his train back to Swindon the small flat felt empty. It was a relief to be alone again – I was so used to being by myself that I found it difficult to relax during prolonged periods of company – yet my thoughts remained with Drew. He was worried about his freelance contract at WHSmith not being renewed. He was 12,000 miles from home. Perhaps I just felt sorry for him.

One week later we had afternoon tea at The Savoy. The fact that Drew was an Australian tourist provided me with an alibi. This time he was more handsome than I had remembered. His boyish grin when he spotted me in the foyer warmed my heart. We went on to see *Don Giovanni* at the Coliseum, and then had supper at the Groucho Club. He had a glass of rosé; I drank a glass of champagne. It was years since I had done so much on a Saturday – or had so much fun. The sex was even better this time round.

It was a novelty to wake up with another person – someone who actually wanted to hold me in his arms. TVP had usually groaned, turned over and gone back to sleep. Drew's strength and warmth made me reluctant to get up but he dragged me off for lunch at the Royal Festival Hall before taking me to 'The Art of Ancient Mexico' exhibition at the Hayward Gallery. I wandered around looking at the other visitors as much as the exhibits. Could they tell Drew and I were lovers? I hoped so. One of the highlights of the show was a Mayan ceremonial death mask made of jade and malachite. Drew bought a postcard of it.

The fact that Drew was a foreigner only really came to matter when he had to get his working visa renewed. Until I met him I shared the same preconceptions and prejudices that most British people have about Australia. It was the land of Rolf Harris, Dame Edna and Skippy the bush kangaroo. The home of good cricket, excellent wine and bad television. A dream holiday destination to which I had never been. Having such a magic far-away homeland made Drew seem exotic – even if he did now live in Swindon. I was not surprised when he said he was thinking of moving.

Ten days after our first date Drew called to say that he had taken 'a unit' in the Jericho area of Oxford. I was delighted. Juxon Street was round the corner from Canal Reach, where the very first episode of *Inspector Morse*, 'The Dead of Jericho', had been shot. The seductive way in which the series portrayed the city had long made me want to live there. Misery in beautiful surroundings was an addictive combination. Morse was as unlucky in love as I was. We were both old before our time.

'Are we going steady now?'

I laughed. Nobody had ever asked me that before. It was typical of courteous, old-fashioned Drew to put it this way. I was ridiculously pleased. I had auditioned three other men who had replied to my ad but, for one reason or a dozen, they had failed.

'Yes, I suppose we are.' I was unsure how I felt about Drew yet I knew that I could trust him. I had no hesitation in calling the electricity board and British Telecom so that he could have power and a telephone in his new home. Someone had to vouch for him.

The next weekend I caught the 11.20 train from Paddington to Oxford. It was packed. I appreciated the space and solitude as I walked along the muddy towpath to Jericho. The golden horse-chestnut leaves in the canal looked like the outstretched hands of drowning men. When Drew opened the front door he flung his arms around me. We were naked in seconds.

Castle Mill House had been designed as student accommodation; each apartment was meant to be shared. The large study/bedroom had two desks, two wardrobes and two single beds. There was an *en suite* kitchen in an alcove and a basic bathroom off the hall. The fridge was filthy. I set about cleaning it while Drew made a late lunch.

The divans, if pushed together, made a double bed of sorts but Drew only had a single duvet. A shopping spree was in order. It was fun bouncing around on all the different beds in the department store. When I suggested Drew join me on a mattress he would grin but shake his head and walk away. We returned to Juxon Street with everything we needed: a couple of lamps, pillows, double sheets and a king-size continental quilt. It was almost time for *Blind Date* when we had finished turning the flat into a home. Drew confessed that he had applied to be on the show and had even been for an interview in London. He was still waiting to hear if he had been chosen. I was amazed. Australians were very popular contestants but surely Drew was too shy to take part? And did he really want a girlfriend? 'Of course not. It's the free holiday I'm after.' We opened a bottle of champagne to celebrate his move. He seemed to be acquiring a taste for it.

I slept very badly that night. The bed was comfortable, the quilt was warm – we had got the highest tog rating available because Drew, as a Queenslander, found the English autumn very cold – and yet, in spite of all our efforts, the room was wrong. The fridge rattled and hummed but the real racket came from Drew. His snoring disturbed me even though I was wearing ear-plugs – as I had done every night since moving to London in 1985. The capital had made me neurotic about noise. Now I could not sleep without them. I was one of those people who needed eight hours of quality sleep each night. If I did not get them I could not function properly. Lack of sleep severely diminished my ability to cope with everyday life. At this stage I viewed each day as an obstacle course to be negotiated: problems not pleasures always seemed to lie ahead. Sleep represented the best means of escape. I wished it were otherwise but it was not – and, as a habitual pessimist, I believed there was nothing I could do about it.

'Turn over!' I prodded him once more.

'Sorry.' He turned on to his side. Ten minutes later he was at it again.

'Drew!'

'I can't help it.' He pulled the duvet over his head. I moved as far away from him as I could, frustration fighting exhaustion. This was never going to work.

Sunday dawned bright and breezy – which was more than could be said for me. I felt as though I had jet-lag. We went for a walk round the centre of Oxford. The Cotswold stone of the colleges glowed yellow in the sharp sunlight. I spotted some familiar faces near the Sheldonian Theatre: it was the crew of *The Mystery of Morse*, a documentary intended to mark what was then supposed to be the final episode of *Inspector Morse*, 'Twilight of the Gods'. I had been a consultant on the programme and, off-camera, conducted the interviews for it. However, I was in no mood to fraternise. We went off in the opposite direction. Drew took me to St Aldate's where the photograph he sent me had been taken. He hunkered down between the same two gravestones and smiled. A moving picture.

After lunch we returned to Castle Mill House to watch 'The Dead of Jericho'.

It is always odd seeing where you are on television: turning it into an electronic image seems to give it an extra validity. An artificial medium creating a greater reality: the cheap paradox of the box.

Drew came with me to the station. I gave him a copy of Dirk Bogarde's novel, *Jericho*, as a parting gift. I did not like to think of him going back by himself through the dark. I called him when I got in. We chatted for about forty minutes. In some ways we seemed to get on better when we were apart. I felt more in control, could think more clearly, when alone. I was becoming increasingly fond of Drew even though he deprived me of sleep. Had I spent so much time alone that I could no longer live with anyone else?

I did my best to let Drew into my life. As his friends were on the other side of the world, mine had to become his. This was not difficult: Drew was far more likeable than me. We went to a Halloween party which, for some reason, had a Wild West theme. My friend and former colleague Elaine had, however, neglected to tell me. Half of *Time Out* were there in cowboy outfits, smashed on margaritas, and, if it was strange for me to see so many old colleagues in one place, it was even odder for them to find me, after all this time, part of a couple. I was proud to be seen with Drew. The novelty of the phrase 'my boyfriend' had not yet worn off. In conversations with friends I had even started to say 'we' instead of 'I'.

Earlier that evening Drew had accompanied me to a library in Welwyn Garden City where, along with the executive producer of *Inspector Morse*, I provided the commentary to a slideshow about the phenomenal success of the series. The idea was to sell a few more copies of my book. Afterwards, a middle-aged couple suggested, in a roundabout way, that Drew and I were, perhaps, a couple too. Drew said nothing. I said 'yes', and realised for the first time that Drew was helping me regain my self-confidence.

David and Tom spent most weekends in deepest Oxfordshire. Their eighteenth-century cottage in Burdrop had three bedrooms so Drew and I could have separate rooms when we went to stay. I had been at school with David but lost touch with him when he went up to Oxford. Years later I discovered that he now lived in Canonbury, just a mile away from Shakespeare Walk. He had met Tom while in Oxford and they had been together ever since. That was how it was supposed to be: you met someone, fell in love, set up home with them and then lived happily ever after. Other people managed to do this, but not me. It could not just be a question of luck.

We took our hosts to Stratford to see John Nettles and Samantha Bond in *The Winter's Tale* at the Royal Shakespeare Theatre. However, it was Richard McCabe as Autolycus, the 'snapper-up of unconsidered trifles', who stole the show. It was good to go out with a couple and, for once, be part of a couple too. It felt as though my life had changed overnight. It had happened so quickly – and the relative ease with which it had made me suspicious. I was so used to things going wrong I hardly dared hope my affair with Drew would last. Would we be together for as long as David and Tom? The following evening, before returning to London, we had a bonfire party, our rockets shattering the black stillness of the valley. So what did David make of Drew? 'He's a lovely boy – when he's not being a spoilt brat.' David never minced his words.

What he said made me think. I always assumed that any disagreement between us was my fault, not Drew's. Most people had to balance the demands of their work and private life. It was a juggling act and I was out of practice. I felt the loss of time and privacy keenly. A sense of backlog, of things to be done piling up, increased the pressure I felt myself to be under. Freelances are always at work, even when they are at home. When Drew left his office he left his work behind and, not unreasonably, wanted to spend his spare time with me. The trouble was, I did not have any spare time. My circle of friends had filled the gap where my other half should have been. Now I had a partner it was a question of widening the circle to let him in. Drew did not seem to understand this. Did he expect me to drop everything and everybody for him?

The crunch came one Saturday when I went to see *The Magic Flute* at the Coliseum with a friend, Mandy. It had been arranged for weeks. Even though it was a matinée perform-ance, I could not get an extra ticket for Drew. He said he would go shopping in the West End and meet us later, so that we could all go back for dinner at Mandy's new flat in Highbury. I could tell he was not happy.

I was looking forward to a friendly, relaxing meal. Mandy had gradually convinced me that there was much more to vegetarian cuisine than penitential nut roasts. That evening she made a spicy casserole of onions, peppers, aubergines, broccoli, courgettes, tomatoes and kidney beans. The conversation flowed along with the wine. I was pleased when Mandy and Henry both let me know how much they liked Drew. 'Forget about his visa running out,' said Mandy. 'Cross that bridge when you come to it. Enjoy yourself. You're very lucky to have met him.'

I was, as usual, starving. I was still going to the gym, slowly increasing my weights, rowing till the sweat poured off me, the old laundry echoing to a chorus of grunts, curses and Annie Lennox: 'Keep Young and Beautiful', 'Walking on Broken Glass' or, the one that really struck a chord, 'Why'. The exercise never got any easier. Some days, when I emerged from the sauna, I could hardly stand up in the shower. The sudden spread of warmth through the entire body, the endorphin rush, almost made the exertion worthwhile. However, I was about to discover that it did not just boost your metabolism. It made you more aggressive as well.

The casserole was delicious. Drew, though, did not think so. He pushed the vegetables round his plate.

'What's the matter? Don't you like it?'

'Yes. Well . . .' He smiled ruefully. 'It's just that I'm allergic to capsicum.'

'Capsicum?'

'Peppers.'

'Oh, you should have said.' Mandy reached for his plate. 'I'll get you something else.'

'No, really. It's all right. I'm not that hungry.'

'Drew, don't tell lies.' I was getting angry. He was letting me down. Mandy had done her best to make him feel welcome. Now, here he was, throwing all her hard work back in her face.

'I am not.'

'Course not. Just like you haven't been sulking all afternoon. I told you. I tried to get you a ticket for the opera but there weren't any left.'

'Mark. It doesn't matter. There's plenty of other stuff to eat.' Mandy got up and went into the kitchen.

'It does matter. You – and I – have got better things to do than run around after his highness.' Mandy's partner, Henry, coughed and refilled our glasses. I was slightly drunk. I was overwrought. I could feel my fury mounting. There was nothing I could do. The sheer strength of it was astonishing. I very rarely lost my temper – I could not even remember the last time it had happened – so the novelty of the sensation added to the drama. Something had to give: Drew. He saw the look in my eyes and stood up. So did I. He moved towards the bathroom, quickly.

'That's right. Why don't you just fuck off?' I paced around the room, my fists clenched. Where had that come from? I was not going to hit him. I would never hit him. I did it again, my hands closing round an invisible crossbar. Perhaps, now that I lifted weights day after day, it had become a habit.

'I'm sorry.' I sat down. I could not stop shaking. Mandy and Henry stared at me. 'I've made a terrible mistake. I'm sorry. We are clearly not meant for each other. I'm sorry you had to see this.'

'I wouldn't have missed it for anything,' said Mandy. 'Poor Drew. I'll put the coffee on. There's *tarte tatin*. Your favourite.'

Drew returned to the table. His face was white. 'Don't worry,' said Henry. 'The tantrum's over.'

'It's not the only thing,' I said. I went to the bathroom and threw up.

We left straight after the coffee. The frost in the air emphasised the chill between us. 'Make it up,' whispered Mandy as I kissed her goodbye. 'Don't be a fool.' It was a bit late for that.

Drew did not say a word on the way back. I walked faster than he did but made no attempt to slow down. I was thinking. As my head cleared I realised that I was afraid of losing him. I was my own worst enemy. The prospect of being trapped in a relationship with a virtual stranger had made me panic. I was the one who usually made all the running. I was not accustomed to being pursued. It had all happened so quickly. Could it really be this easy? Was Drew the one for me? I hardly knew him – and, more to the point, I hardly knew myself. I could either break the whole thing off and retreat into bitter isolation or apologise and stumble on towards some kind of understanding. Which was it going to be?

When we got in I set about making some camomile tea. Drew came into the kitchen and put his arms around me. I burst into tears.

'I'm sorry. It's all my fault. I didn't want to hurt you. I love you.' The three little words just came out. Was it true? I wasn't sure. Probably.

'I love you too.'

'Really? Even after tonight?'

'Even after tonight. But if you ever hit me that will be it. Believe me, the first time will be the last time.'

'I won't. I promise. I don't want to lose you.' I rested my head on his shoulder. 'It's all happened so fast though. We hardly know each other.'

'It only takes a second to fall in love. I think I know you pretty well.'

After my sleepless stay in Oxford Drew had agreed to spend each night in London on the sofa-bed in the living room. Nevertheless, I often woke in the morning to find him snuggled up next to me. The day after my outburst I was relieved to sense him sneaking into my bed at dawn. A couple of weeks later, back in the stalls, having pulled a few strings, I watched Drew wait for the Queen of the Night to hit her top F.

We celebrated my thirtieth birthday at the Groucho Club. I had been dreading the watershed all year but could hardly ignore the day itself. The sixteenth of November 1992 was a Monday, so, on the previous Saturday, sixteen of us gathered in the club's Bloomsbury Room. I plied them with champagne; they showered me with gifts. What made the most impression, however, was Drew's birthday card. In addition to copying out the entire lyrics to Gene Pitney's 'Something's Gotten Hold of My Heart', Drew had neatly printed: 'The song on the opposite page actually sounds really nice when sung and I should probably let you hear it. At the moment you mean an awful lot to me, even if I don't always show and/or say it. Anyway, what can I say, the big three O. Let's hope we all see thrice thirty and more years yet as the future unfolds. Happy birthday my love. The adventure has just begun.'

After dinner someone suggested that everybody take it in turns to say something about me. Howard explained how he and I first met: as thirteen-year-olds seated together in third-form History. Geoff from *Time Out* revealed why he had originally chosen me to work as holiday relief in the film section from the hundreds of other applicants: anybody who had once worked on the sweet counter in Woolworth's deserved a break. And Pascal, as mischievous as ever, paid tribute to my 'virility'. On our last, drunken, evening at Le Lac I had finally dared to go skinny-dipping. Swimming alone with him in the warm moonlight was intensely erotic. The freezing water had done nothing to cool my ardour. I got my own back when it was my turn to say something about all of them.

The love and affection demonstrated by my friends touched me deeply. I was glad Drew was there to share it – even if he was finding out rather too much about me. For once I felt accepted. We did not usually do this kind of thing: we were more likely to hug each other than discuss our innermost feelings. I was afraid my sister Linda would deduce that I was gay but, if she had any suspicions, she kept them to herself. I did want to tell her. However, when, still reeling from my first gay experience at university, I had told her that I had been to bed with another boy, she had burst into tears and begged me never to do it again. Her reaction had upset me, but then, she was only sixteen at the time. I blamed the parents.

My sister had left her husband Craig behind in Lancaster and come down to London with a friend instead. As I could not afford to put them up in a hotel, they had to stay with me. I thought it important that at least one member of my family came to the party. It seemed only right to let the girls have my room. I would shift on to the sofa-bed but Drew's snoring, and our sex, meant there was no way we could share it. He would have to sleep somewhere else. I felt guilty about making him homeless. Alex, however, said he could stay at his place. 'It will have to be on a sofa, though – unless Greg lets him sleep with him. You wouldn't mind, would you?' Greg was Alex's new lodger – apparently gorgeous, and another Aussie to boot.

When Drew rang to wish me happy birthday on the Monday – and to say how much he loved me – he did not mention his night in Sotheby Road. Three days later he was back there for Alex's twenty-ninth birthday party.

Alex was, of course, drunk by the time we arrived. So was everyone else.

'Glad you could make it.' He placed my present on a pile of unopened ones. 'The booze is in the kitchen.' He handed

Drew his empty glass. 'Fill me up, sweetie. You know where to go.'

'Champagne?'

'Yes, please.' Alex and I spoke in unison. Drew rolled his eyes and disappeared.

'Good. You'll never guess who's here. Steven. Don't look like that. Come and say hello.'

I followed him as he jostled his way through the crowd. Nobody could have this many friends. I hardly recognised anyone. We climbed the steep stairs to the upper half of the living room where, even though it was late autumn, the French windows that led to the roof terrace were wide open. Someone was letting off rockets.

'Hello.' I turned round. Here, finally, was a familiar face. 'Long time no see.'

'Well, your luck's just run out.' He was as handsome as ever and yet I felt nothing for him. I had once been in love with Steven for more than two years and yet, during all that time, we had never gone to bed: sex, in fact, was the one thing that we had not done together. He had wanted friendship; I had wanted romance. He, as usual, had got his own way. It was the same old story: if I loved someone they did not love me.

Alex had never loved Steven but they had slept together for a while. That was how I met Steven: Alex tried to pass him on to me. I was often grateful for his cast-offs, whether they were items of clothing, furniture or people. Steven, though, would only sleep with men whom he considered to be better-looking than him. He was fortunate, in those early days of

Aids, that he had a very high opinion of himself. Unrequited love is both painful and unhealthy; it nearly drove me out of my mind. However, I only decided to stop seeing Steven when he rang me up in a complete rage and harangued me for twenty minutes. My crime? Sending him a dozen red roses on his birthday.

'Here we are.' Drew appeared at my elbow. 'Where's Alex?'

I nodded towards the terrace, but added, 'Don't bother. He's had too much already. This gentleman will take it off your hands.' I introduced Steven and, while they made small talk, watched the partygoers below yelling in each other's faces. I really was not interested in Steven any more. As Proteus had declared, at the theatre earlier in the evening: 'Even as one heat another heat expels/Or as one nail by strength drives out another,/So the remembrance of my former love/Is by a newer object quite forgotten.'

'He's lovely,' said Steven. Drew was now speaking to someone else. They could not take their eyes off him. 'He'll make you far happier than I ever could.'

'I know. Still with John?'

'Yup.'

'So there you are.' Alex threw his arms round our shoulders. 'Have you two kissed and made up?' Steven looked at me. I looked at him. Alex pushed our heads together. 'No tongues!'

We pecked each other on both cheeks. I suddenly felt tired. I went over to Drew and put my arm round his waist. The man who was chatting him up gave me the gay once-over:

groin, face, feet, groin. That tell-tale flick of the eyeballs always made me squirm. Self-recognition? Self-hate? I could not be bothered to decide. 'Let's go.'

As we reached the front door someone tapped Drew on the shoulder.

'Leaving so soon?'

'This is Greg,' said Drew. He went out on to the landing.

'You must be Mark. I've heard a lot about you.' He was very handsome.

'All bad, I hope.' We shook hands.

'No, mate. Alex thinks the world of you.' He nodded towards Drew. 'Better not keep the sheila waiting.'

We held hands in the minicab. It was too dark for the driver to see.

3

CRUISING

I took Drew to Nice for his birthday. We were both glad to get away.

Three days earlier, on 1 December, I received an early-morning wake-up call from a policeman. The upstairs flat had been burgled during the night – while the whole house had been in bed. The comings and goings in the hall had so disturbed me that I had eventually put down my book and got up to peep out of my own, internal, front door. The man I saw disappearing down the steps had made off with the tele-vision, video recorder and answering machine. I had assumed he was a friend of the couple above and gone back to bed. It was not my fault they had been foolish enough to leave their door unlocked. Nor had they bothered to double-lock the front door, which I always did. It had apparently remained open all night.

It was not my fault but, because I worked at home, it was

left to me to have the locks changed and the new keys cut. Two days later, writing an article on *Inspector Morse* for the *Daily Mirror*, my desk started shaking. Someone was trying to kick their way into the house next door. I called the police: by the time all the details had been taken, another colour television was halfway down twilit Shakespeare Walk. Neither thief was ever caught. Meanwhile, back in Oxford, Drew had been warned that a prowler was on the loose in Jericho. We both expected to return from France to ransacked flats.

The thought of losing personal property was bad enough, but what really worried me was the idea of someone invading my private space. The only recurrent nightmare I had ever suffered was that of waking up with a stranger standing over me. It rarely occurred more than once a month. Recently, however, it had been happening with increasing frequency and intensity. I could hear the man – it was always a man – breaking down the door. I could feel the bed shaking. I could not move. I would wake up, drenched in sweat, staring into the darkness, holding my breath, convinced there was someone in the room. It took a long time for my heartbeat to slow down.

The eighth of December, Drew's twenty-eighth birthday, was a Tuesday – which he would have to spend at work in Swindon. So on the previous Friday we caught an afternoon flight from Heathrow to Nice. We touched down in pouring rain. Vanessa Paradis cheered us up singing 'Be My Baby' on the radio in the taxi. Knowing Drew's views on cabbies – he earned twice as much as me, yet when a taxi-driver once mistakenly gave him a £20 note instead of a fiver in his change, he kept it because the cabbie had overcharged him by 10p – and the extortionate rates on the Riviera, I paid. The Beau Rivage was quiet and comfortable. We drank the champagne from the minibar and put both mattresses to the test. They passed.

We had twin beds because I had been too lily-livered to book a double. I could just imagine the bellboy's leers and sneers when he showed us to our room. Besides, I did not want Drew snoring in my ear. Of course, the extra few feet between us made little difference. Perhaps, given time, I would get used to the noise. My maternal grandmother had put up with my grandfather's apocalyptic snoring for nearly forty years. When his beloved Capstan Full Strength eventually took their toll she could not sleep for the silence.

However, it was not sound but light that woke me the next morning. I did not know where I was. Sunshine streamed through a gap in the heavy, ornate curtains. Drew was still in dreamland. I watched him slumber on, pleased to see his familiar face. I felt lucky to have woken up next to him. I wanted to kiss him but did not want to disturb him.

After croissants and coffee in bed we set off to explore Nice. The Promenade des Anglais was virtually deserted. The Bay of Angels reflected the clear, blue sky overhead. We took it in turns to take each other's photograph. Drew was a magician with the camera. The picture he took of me outside the Hotel Negresco immediately became my favourite when I collected it from Boots the following week. I looked slim, young, fit and happy — it was as if Drew saw me the way I wanted to be seen. We clicked.

We strolled round the flower market, up to the castle, and down to the old port for lunch. A French naval vessel was docked in the harbour. It was decked out in bunting for some sort of Open Day. A group of ratings kicked their heels at the bottom of the gangplank. They looked very cute in their tight-fitting navy blue uniforms. When they saw us watching them they waved their red-pompommed berets and shouted something. A-level French had not prepared me for flirting with sailors. They were probably just offering to give us a guided tour of the ship but I was not going to take any chances. We were heavily outnumbered. Anyway, the whole idea of two Brits being shown round a man-of-war by a handful of French cadets was just too camp. We waved back and, somewhat reluctantly, moved on. Theatrical groaning gave way to laughter.

'Would you like to go to a sauna?' The question stopped me in my tracks.

'What, now? Here in Nice? Is there one?'

'Of course there is. It's not far from here.'

'How do you know?'

'I looked it up in *Spartacus*.' *Spartacus* is a gay travel guide that caters to those with wanderlust.

'I've never been to a sauna.' Drew looked at me. The sun made him squint.

'I thought you said there was one at the gym.'

'There is — and it's the size of a telephone kiosk. Any more than three and it's like the Black Hole of Calcutta.' I carried on walking. 'Do you want to go?'

'It might be fun. We're in a foreign country. Nobody knows us. We might meet a few sailor boys.'

'Okay. Lead on, Macduff.' He pulled a photocopied page out of his pocket and studied it. 'It's called Le Sept.'

The place, down a quiet side-street, was easy enough to find. We rang the buzzer and were immediately admitted to a tiny vestibule. The window of a cubby-hole slid open and a fat bald man said 'hello'. Not '*bonjour*', but 'hello'. We obviously did not look French. We handed over the requisite amount of francs and received a couple of keys in return. A second door buzzed open. We were in.

The butterball came out of his office and gave us both a threadbare green towel. He led us through a lounge area into the changing-room. Dark eyes followed us lazily. I began to feel nervous. We undressed quickly, wrapped the towels round our waists and then stowed our clothes in metal lockers.

'What do we do now?' I whispered. I really did not want to be here. The thought of being surrounded by a gang of semi-naked Frenchmen was exciting in theory but terrifying in practice.

'Let's go exploring.' Drew smiled. 'Don't look so worried. I'll protect you.'

The showers — six metal roses all in a row — were empty. Opposite them were doors to the steam room and sauna. At the end of the corridor steps led down into a Jacuzzi large enough to hold an entire football team. However, at this time, it contained just three men. One of them was floating on his back. His circumcised cock bobbed about in the bubbles.

Spectators could, if they wished, sit on benches around the sides.

The first floor had been converted into a maze of cabins. Most were unoccupied but in some of them men reclined on single mattresses playing with themselves, waiting for someone to join them. One hairy-chested guy waved at Drew and opened his towel.

'God knows why this place is called Le Sept. I haven't seen a seven-incher yet.'

'Shh!'

The whole sauna was eerily quiet. Hot and dimly lit, it was like the nocturnal house at the zoo. There were plenty of strange creatures here as well. The clientele featured far more sad sacks than six-packs. Old queens gazed longingly at young studs. The latter tended to keep their towels wrapped round themselves. The former were more brazen and either carried their towel or slung it over their shoulders, any sense of modesty just a distant memory. Their balls hung as low as their expectations.

'Now what? Do we just keep wandering around? I thought you wanted a break from sightseeing.'

'Let's try the steam room.'

I let Drew go first. It was difficult to see where you were going until your eyes had adapted to the gloom. We groped our way across the room and sat down on the plastic ledge that ran around the walls. It was suffocatingly hot. Still, the steam did feel good as it gently opened up your pores. My towel was sopping wet. I realised now that I should have hung it up outside like Drew. However, I had been too scared to enter the chamber of horrors stark-naked. Besides, my cock had shrivelled in fear.

We were, I guessed, in the company of seven other people. They could have been Greek gods or German dogs: it was impossible to tell from the blurred outlines. That, presumably, was the point of these establishments: they held out the prospect of sex to anyone and everyone. Somebody was using poppers, amyl nitrate. A sudden flurry of activity opposite was followed by a grunt. The unmistakable smell of spunk filled the air. I felt sick.

'I'm going to cool off in the showers.'

'Okay. I'll be out in a minute.'

There was one other person showering, a muscular, middle-aged man with lightning zigzags tattooed on each forearm. He watched as I removed my towel then looked away. I waited for the water to warm up slightly and then stepped beneath its needle jets. I closed my eyes and let all the sweat stream away. A pair of hands gripped my buttocks.

'Everyone else turn you down then?' I thought it was Drew. It was not. The hands slid round to my groin. I opened my eyes and saw blue lightning. My companion in the shower now had a hard-on. I tried to look suitably impressed, smiled apologetically and grabbed my towel.

There was no sign of Drew. I went down to the Jacuzzi and sat on one of the benches. The pool was empty. The coast was clear. I might as well give it a go.

The churning water, a thousand licking tongues, jiggled your genitals – by no means an unpleasant sensation. It was too hot though, and the chlorine made your eyes sting. Soon pins and needles started shooting down my arms. I was going to faint. I staggered out, sat down and stuck my head between my knees.

The passing trade began to pick up. Saturday afternoon was clearly peak time. I stayed where I was on the sidelines and began to enjoy the occasional piece of scenery. Whenever my mother saw a naked man on television she would invariably say: 'Once you've seen one you've seen them all.' How wrong she was. Peggy Lee's 'Pass Me By' popped into my head: 'Contemplatin' nature can be fascinatin' . . . if you don't happen to like it pass me by.' I could not help smiling. Nobody smiled back.

I was not surprised. Pornography depends on po-faces. Sex, for this mob, was a serious business. A single laugh could destroy the carefully created illusion, reveal the ludicrousness inherent in all such situations. These naked men drifting through the shadows down here, flitting from cell to cell up there, were all seeking to fulfil the fantasies peddled by pornographers. Surely it would have been easier to stay at home and, just for a change, wank with the other hand?

Why had Drew brought me here? Three months ago I would not have dared to enter a gay sauna. My new-found confidence remained fragile: some of the bodies on display today proved that I still had a long, long way to go. I was hardly God's gift. Perhaps I was being naïve expecting someone like Drew to settle for me and me alone. I found it hard to believe that someone like Drew was interested in someone like me. Perhaps I had never had a long-term relationship because my novelty wore off all too soon. I had the sudden urge to talk to him about this. Where the hell was he?

At the top of the narrow stairs I was greeted by a scene straight out of Hieronymus Bosch. Each cabin offered a variation on a theme: to walk along the narrow passage was like surfing through a dozen adult cable channels. Only embarrassment made me look away: it was rude to stare. Any of the writhing bodies could have belonged to Drew but I somehow doubted it. Still, I now knew that three into one *would* go.

What I had witnessed was fascinating rather than erotic: more like maggots squirming in a dish than men making love. How did they achieve such abandon? Did the fact that they were being watched turn them on? It was, I supposed, all a question of performance.

I went back downstairs and decided to have a final shower. Perhaps Drew had already got dressed. A curly-haired boy was soaping another's back in the showers. He let his hands slowly slip down to caress the chunky white arse. It was Drew's. The boy, who had a great tan, saw me but did not stop. I wanted to leave, to leave them to it, but I was transfixed.

Drew turned round. Our eyes met. He stood there while the teenage wet-dream continued to rub himself against him. Someone else came into the showers. I returned to the locker-room and dried myself with my T-shirt.

'I wasn't doing anything,' said Drew as we walked back to the hotel.

'No . . . but you weren't doing anything to stop him either.'

'I didn't have a hard-on.'

'God knows why. You must have felt his up against you. You lucky bastard.' We both laughed. 'Don't worry about it.'

It had been the sexiest moment of the afternoon. The French had given us the word voyeurism, so where better to first sample its live joys than the back streets of Nice? The city appeared so clean, open and modern at first sight, but it had its hidden parts, its dark and dirty corners. Perhaps Drew was not as innocent as he seemed. He had a history too.

Back at the Beau Rivage I felt so ill I had to go to bed. Chlorine poisoning could have caused the headache and nausea but such symptoms were more likely to have been the result of chronic dehydration. I drank bottle after bottle of mineral water and lay there while Drew ran his fingers through my hair.

'I'm sorry. I knew you didn't want to go but I thought you might like it.'

'I wouldn't have missed it for the world.'

As usual my flippancy was a defence mechanism. I considered myself reasonably broad-minded but some of the antics in those public rooms had shocked me. Watching porn in private is not the same as experiencing it in real life. And, to cap it all, I had suddenly seen Drew in a whole new light. Was prudishness a sign of encroaching middle age?

'Were you jealous?'

'I should have been, but I wasn't really. It was odd, though, seeing you with someone else. My first thought was: get your hands off my property. Then I got turned on. You were pretty horny . . . for a pair of sluts.'

'Thanks a lot. Maybe we'll have a threesome one day. You know, to spice things up. We're bound to be bored with each other after a couple of years.' Somehow I did not think that my novelty value would last that long.

'So we'll still be together then?'

'Hopefully.' He kissed me. 'Try to sleep.'

I felt much better when I woke up – and very hungry. We had dinner in a cosy Italian restaurant – candles stuck in Chianti bottles, black-and-white photographs of Naples on the walls – and, not daring to hold hands, walked back along the promenade. I was happy to be taking my boyfriend home to bed.

On the flight back to London Drew asked me to accompany him on a cruise round the Caribbean. I thought he was joking.

'I'd love to, but I can't afford it.'

'I know that. It would be my treat.'

'When would you want to go?' I still did not believe him.

'We set sail on the second of January and return to Fort Lauderdale on the twelfth.'

'We?'

'I booked my place months ago – before I met you. As things stand I'll be sharing the cabin with a stranger. I'd much rather the other person was you.'

'So would I.' I had never been to the Caribbean. 'Are you sure about this?'

'Absolutely.'

One telephone call and my place on the cruise was

confirmed. It was clearly meant to be. I celebrated by going to the gym and managed to do ten minutes on the rowing machine for the first time. Your muscles ached and stiffened even if you missed a single work-out; the nagging sensation only served to increase your sense of guilt.

I was also feeling guilty about not spending Christmas with Drew. I was going home to my family in Lancaster as usual, but he was not flying back to Cairns. He decided to take a trip to Disneyland Paris instead. He already knew I would never accompany him there. He was accustomed to travelling alone – and had been prepared to share a cabin with a total stranger. His self-sufficiency and self-confidence were partly what attracted me to him: the paradox was that such qualities made me want to look after him. He was far more trusting than me.

In the meantime I had a lot of work to do before running away to sea. Freelances do not get paid when they go on holiday. My best birthday present turned out to be a telephone call from a friend who had once worked in the *Time Out* television section – was I interested in previewing some programmes for the *Sunday Times*? The biggest problem was finding out what was going to be broadcast between 28 December 1992 and 2 January 1993 – and then getting hold of the videotapes. If *Merry Christmas Mr Bean* was fun, *Stars in Their Eyes: Elvis Special* was not. The new year saw the start of the new television franchises so it was goodbye to TV-am and Thames and hello to GMTV and Carlton. I also had to fly to Dublin to interview the cast and crew of *The Snapper*, the second part of Roddy Doyle's Barrytown trilogy. The assignment had not come from a glossy magazine but a PR company that needed someone to compile the press-pack, the bumf handed out to journalists when a film is released. Mindful of my increasing overdraft, I had swallowed my pride and accepted the work with gratitude.

I saw Drew whenever I could. We laughed ourselves silly at *Strictly Ballroom* in the dark depths of the Renoir; loved and hated Ken Russell's *Iolanthe* at the Coliseum; adopted the catchphrase of the Australian trio performing *The Complete Works of William Shakespeare (Abridged)* at the Arts Theatre ('maybe, maybe not'); and goggled at Patricia Routledge bursting out all over the National in *Carousel*. The three months since I had met Drew had been the most hectic of my life. He transformed the stay-at-home me into a gadabout: 'It's not against the law to enjoy yourself, you know.' It was exciting and exhausting. Drew saw the world from a completely different angle: he challenged me to justify my point of view whether we were discussing the American invasion of Somalia or the fire at Windsor Castle (he naturally preferred to be called an ardent royalist rather than a craven colonial). His energy and enthusiasm were infectious.

I thought I was getting better at juggling the demands of work and play, of my friends and my lover. Drew, however, sent me a cartoon torn from a recent copy of the *Spectator*. It showed a couple standing by the Thames in London: '1. How many friends have you got? A hundred and thirty-four. 2. How often do you see them? All the time. 3. That gives you no time for yourself . . . I don't need any time for myself. It's all for my friends. 4. Why did you reply to my ad in the personal column?' If he was dissatisfied, though, why did he continue to pursue me? I still could not work out what he saw in me. He was a kind, Christian computer programmer; I was a cynical older hack.

He called at 9.30 on Christmas morning. Linda answered the telephone; she and Craig always came for breakfast on the 25th in the same way that our grandmother always came to stay. The Sanderson Christmas followed an unbreakable routine.

'It's Drew. He sounds a long way away.'

'He's in Paris.'

'Lucky thing.' She handed me the receiver.

'Hello?'

'Merry Christmas!'

'Merry Christmas. Thanks for the presents. They're great. I think you're too good for me.'

It was true. I had opened his gift before taking the train up to Lancaster. I had had too much to carry as it was. He had covered the box in paper decorated with holly and topped it off with a homemade bow. Ten years on, I still use it to keep receipts in. It is strange how the most disposable of objects can become an enduring part of your life. Back then the box contained a bar of strawberry soap in the shape of a butterfly, a pencil eraser in the shape of an aeroplane, a framed photograph of the two of us taken by a friendly passer-by in Nice and *The Little Book of Hugs*, all individually wrapped. The book was revoltingly sentimental, took less than ten minutes to read, and yet I was touched. The photograph, in its mahogany frame, lent our relationship an air of permanence that both pleased and frightened me.

I did not like to think of him all by himself amid the synthetic bonhomie of a freezing theme park: whether eating over-priced burgers or being strapped in roller-coasters with screaming kids, he was being taken for a ride.

'We must spend next Christmas together.'

'Definitely.'

It was not to be. The following year the physical distance between us could not have been greater.

I had always thought of cruise ships as floating Butlin's camps, the preserve of well-off pensioners who whiled away the hours between banquets playing bowls or simply shuffling along the decks on their Zimmer frames. The *Sky Princess* had sailed across television screens around the world. It provided the exterior shots of the liner in a seaborne soap called *The Love Boat*. As we left the quayside in Fort Lauderdale, throwing free streamers at the people down below, its theme music came blaring out of the Tannoy: 'Lurve is exciting and new / Come aboard, we're expecting you . . .' 'Oh gross!' said Drew.

I had decided to leave my embarrassment at home. Cruising was naff and there was nothing I could do about it. After all, everybody – the honeymooners from Des Moines, the retirees from Bournemouth, the cruise junkies from New York and the novices from 'Old London Town', as the Americans insisted on calling it – was in the same boat and would be for the next twelve days. Our cover story was that I was a journalist and Drew was my photographer: 'Get one of that sign, Drew. SLOW SPEED – MANATEE AREA.' I never expected to actually write about the trip.

We had got off to a smooth enough start. The flight from Gatwick to Miami had arrived on time on New Year's Day. However, there was no one from P & O waiting for us in the arrivals lounge as promised. We took a cab to the nearby Sofitel Hotel. It had no record of our reservation. The lobby was packed with irate holiday-makers. After a very long wait, the only room they could offer us was one with a kingsize double bed.

'Sir, is there a problem?' asked the receptionist. Her sense of humour appeared to have checked out long ago.

'Grown men don't usually share beds in Britain.'

'That's not what I've heard.'

We took the room, retrieved our swimming costumes and went down to the outdoor pool. It was January but the air was hot and humid. Bemused faces peered down at us from the tower of net-curtained windows. Jet after jet screamed off into the lurid sunset.

Twenty-four hours later we were sailing into another sunset. This time the sky was an angry mass of black and orange. The tugboat *Captain Nelson* towed us into the teeth of a gale. Plastic recliners skidded across the sun-deck and flipped into the sloshing pool. Waitresses struggled to keep their balance. And the calypso band played on.

The wind increased in strength as we passed the beachside condos and reached the open sea. A few bored residents waved good riddance from their balconies. We did not care. It was not cold. We were virtually alone on the top deck. Most people had taken shelter in the lounges below. My longish hair took on a life of its own and made Drew giggle. He taped the Medusan spectacle with his camcorder. He spent most of the cruise with one eye pressed to its viewfinder whether we were in a helicopter over St Lucia or on jet-skis in the Bahamas.

'Why don't you experience something at first sight for a change?'

'I promised I'd send a tape to my parents. You'll be glad I did this one day.'

'Okay, guys. Closer together.' One of the ubiquitous ship's photographers, wearing the regulation pink shirt and white shorts, thrust his Nikon at us. Drew kept on recording. I knew instinctively that he fancied the happy snapper.

'Come on, come on, put the camera down. Make with the cheesy grins.' He was only doing his job. Drew did as he was told. We smiled. There was a flash and the photographer was off in search of his next victims. His pictures, and those of his colleagues, would be on sale the next day. Being on board meant being in shot. The ship was a maritime mall with a captive clientele.

To begin with it was more like starting boarding school than being on holiday. Suitcases and trunks blocked the corridors. You did not know where to go or what to do – but all the older boys did. We had to queue to be assigned our places at dinner. We had to attend a lifeboat drill. Even the atmosphere was the familiar one of vague excitement mixed with dread.

Our cabin, however, was better than the study-bedrooms to which I was accustomed. It was situated on the Lido Deck, the highest level of accommodation, and designated a 'mini-suite': this meant there was a living area with a couch, desk, coffee table and wall-mounted TV, as well as a sleeping area with two single beds. There was a large window instead of a porthole, but no balcony. The room may have been very brown, worn and tasteless, yet it soon felt like a home from home. The distant thunder of the engines even masked Drew's snoring. Slightly.

The bathroom featured a vacuum toilet. 'Don't flush it while you're sitting on it,' said the maid, 'otherwise you'll lose your bowels.' The stool in the shower apparently suggested the advanced age of most passengers until I felt the ship roll beneath me. So that was why there was a carpet on the wall above the couch. I should have known better. *The Poseidon Adventure* had been on enough times.

There was a roll in both our gaits when we went down for dinner. Drew, having ignored US Customs regulations, produced a bottle of Dom Pérignon from his suitcase to toast our maiden voyage. He was full of surprises. During the flight to Miami he served up the last of a Christmas cake I had given him. Why had he bothered to bring it? Was it a reproach? 'I wanted to share it with you.' We shared the champagne and discovered that two people could just about fit in a single berth.

We were the last people to join our table. Five Canadian women and the ship's doctor awaited us. 'Yes, madam, the *Sky Princess* is a big ship but you can still be sea-sick on her. There's a heavy swell tonight. The Captain's already ordered the stabilisers to be deployed. All portholes have had their storm shutters closed.' Drew did not take the news well.

When I saw the circle of grim faces round Table 155 I wanted to run back and order room service, but then I read the menu. Pan-fried fillet of Mahi Mahi Buccaneer sounded interesting – which was more than could be said of our fellow guests. They were a threesome and a twosome. June, Joan and Shirley were amiable matrons from Montreal in search of good food and a good rest. Kate and Sally from Toronto were our age and desperately seeking sex. Drew, gallant as ever, responded to their flirting but only succeeded in disappointing Kate. In the end she consoled herself with one of our Italian waiters. It was hard to say who was more jealous: me or the miserable Sally.

The doctor was our saviour. He was British and immediately saw how things were between myself and Drew. I could see the boredom beneath his bronzed skin, sense him nerving himself for yet another endless round of gourmet meals and gormless chat. It was part of his job description to dine with prospective patients and, as it happened, Drew would soon be a regular at his surgery. He seemed to enjoy our sparring matches. It was certainly dull when duty kept him away from the table.

*

St Martin was the first port of call. Drew had booked an excursion to each of the islands on our itinerary. He loved islands. His favourite place on the planet was Coochiemudlo Island off the coast of Brisbane. A couple of his friends had a house on it. 'I'll take you there one day. You'll love it.' There was something childlike about his passion for islands and the boats that took you to them. It stemmed partly from the fact that he was a distant relative of Captain Henry Morgan, the English privateer. When he was young, his family had lived for a while in Jamaica, Morgan's old bolt-hole, in a villa over-looking Montego Bay. Drew's horizons were wider than mine – and yet I think islands appealed to him because of their self-containedness. They were havens in a sea of troubles.

Orient Bay was on the north-east coast of St Martin, on the French side of the island. 'Aha!' said the doctor, when we told him where we were going. 'You won't need your Speedos there.' I had never been to a naturist beach. After lunch Drew and I left our party and wandered along the sand to where clothing appeared to be optional. It was a warm, overcast day, and there had already been a couple of showers, but rain made no difference when you were swimming in the Caribbean. Half a dozen naked people were lying on the beach. They raised their heads as we passed. I was glad that I was wearing my Ray-Bans: they let you stare without seeming to do so. Butterflies fluttered in my stomach. We found a quiet spot and sat down. I slipped off my trunks.

'Coming for a paddle?'

Drew shook his head. 'No. I don't feel too good.'

'What's the matter?'

'Think I'm getting a cold. I'll sit here and watch.'

'Well, get your kit off then.'

'Somebody might come along.'

'Suit yourself.' I could not chicken out now. I strolled as nonchalantly as I could down to the water's edge. I did not dare turn round to see if anyone was looking, just plunged into the waves and headed for a pontoon that was moored about a hundred yards out. The sense of freedom was exhilarating. I could not believe I was doing this. In less than six months I had become less fat and more fit. I was undergoing a sea-change.

It took me longer than expected to reach the pontoon. I hauled myself on to it and sat there panting, marvelling at the warmth of the air on my skin. This was the life. I stood up and waved at Drew. He was not the only one who waved back. The windows of a low-rise restaurant, hidden behind a bank of sand dunes, were dotted with faces. I should have stood my ground, enjoyed my moment of unexpected glory, but did not. I jumped straight back into the sea and came up spluttering. The middle of nowhere is hard to find.

I swam slowly round the pontoon a couple of times then headed for the beach. I tugged my cock to give it some heft, then staggered out of the breakers and plodded up the slope to my towel. Drew put his camcorder down. 'Your parents will love that.' I did not mind being caught on camera. I hated being caught out though – it was easier to change the shape of your body than alter your mental make-up.

*

Drew took to his bed when we returned to the *Sky Princess*. I went exploring. The equipment in the gym used compressed air instead of weights for safety reasons. The room was empty. So was the sauna. The cinema, in the bowels of the ship, was showing *Sister Act*. A 'Trivial Pursuit Team Challenge' was under way in the Piano Lounge. You could play 'Family Feud' in the Show Lounge or join Angela in making artificial carnations in the Veranda Lounge. I went to the Rainbow Lounge and ordered the cocktail of the day, Lady of Paradise: peach schnapps, triple sec, strawberry liqueur and cream. According to 'Princess Patter', the daily newsletter, Owen, 'the Yorkshire poet' (Wilfred was born in Shropshire), had immortalised this 'heavenly blend' with the words 'One sip . . . was like an angel crying on my tongue.' 'Crying' was not quite right.

God, I was bored. As I passed the Purser's Office once again I spotted something of interest. One of the junior officers, his tan made deeper by his dashing white uniform, was chatting to an older colleague. Our eyes met. His were puppy-dog brown. I smiled. He smiled. I moved on.

He was called Chip. I saw a lot more of him over the next few days as Drew succumbed to flu. We fell into a ritual. Drew would drag himself out of bed to go on an island tour, make a sandcastle on the beach while I swam in the warm, clear sea, then, on our return to the ship, go straight back to bed. At first I stayed with him, reading or snoozing as well, but I soon got cabin fever. I took my Discman to the sun deck and, even though I was wearing factor 15, got burned. 'Lobster city!' was Drew's only comment. The CD cases carry the lotion stains to this day.

The doctor gave Drew special treatment but could do nothing about his failing sense of humour. Even when in the best of health Drew lacked the ability to laugh at himself. I was 'mean' if I teased him, no matter how affectionately.

I was lonely. Apart from the odd pair of newly-weds, most of the passengers were at least twenty years older than me. I spotted one gay couple, thirtysomething Americans who were clearly devoted to each other. One of the men had purple blotches on his face and arms: the tell-tale signs of Kaposi's sarcoma. I never saw the lovers again.

The crew proved to be as stratified as the ship on which they served. The Captain was British. His officers were either fellow countrymen or Americans. The waiters were Italian, the kitchen staff were Filipino and the boilermen Bangladeshi. 'You have to be used to heat to work in the engine room,' said the doctor. 'It's not a pleasant job. Most of them don't see daylight from one end of a cruise to the other. It can send a man over the edge – literally. We often lose someone off the back of the ship at night. They just can't take any more.' Suddenly the Grand Marnier soufflé did not taste so good.

It was against strict regulations to fraternise with passengers. At the end of his shift Chip would change out of his uniform then meet me by the running track on the top deck. It was usually deserted. The roar from the giant funnels made it impossible to eavesdrop. To begin with we just chatted, but it was obvious to both of us what was going to happen. I had never been to bed with an American, let alone a sexy brat from Beverly Hills. His zip code was actually 90210.

Sunday began with a stupid row. I felt awful. Drew's coughing – and a mosquito – had kept me awake for most of the night. He, however, had woken up feeling much better and planned to go to an aerobics class after he had been to church. I went to the gym, listened to some music on the sun-deck, then had brunch. Early in the afternoon Chip smuggled me into his cabin. His room-mate was working.

Chip was twenty-one. He had puppy fat as well as puppy-dog eyes. It must have been quite some time since he went surfing in Malibu. His flesh was tanned but there was too much of it. Richard Gere wore a similar uniform in *An Officer and a Gentleman* but he looked a lot better than this when he took it off. Chip rolled over and presented a large hairy bottom for inspection. This was not how it was supposed to be. I no longer wished to be in this position. I had to get out.

'What's the matter?'

'I'm sorry. I'm sorry. I can't do this to Drew.' This would not be the last time I used Drew as a pretext for low behaviour. And it was not even true. I had lost my erection because the fantasy had crumbled, not because I had suddenly been overcome with guilt. Drew and I were not married. I had yet to commit myself to him: when I did, I would be faithful. I had no doubt about that. I got up.

'Shit. I knew this would happen. Mark, I really like you. Don't go.'

'I've got to. This is wrong.' I put on my boxer shorts.

'Please stay.' He started to cry. 'I love you.'

'No you don't. You just think you do.'

'I'll tell Drew.'

I laughed. 'Oh yeah? And do you like your job?'

'You wouldn't do that to me.'

'Try me.' I sat down on the edge of the bed. 'Look, let's not leave it like this. We can still be friends.' I tried to touch him but he turned away.

'I've got plenty of friends.' His disappointment turned to anger. 'Oh, go on then. Fuck off back to your wife.'

As Sunday was to be spent entirely at sea we had booked a visit to the bridge. When they heard of our plans Kate and Sally did the same. An officer showed us the various controls and explained what all the dials meant. We studied the radar, examined the rudder-angle indicator and learned what the bow thruster did. The apparatus seemed disconcertingly primitive. Lesson over, the four of us were allowed to go outside and admire the view.

The inevitable photo session ensued. Drew wanted me to take a picture of him with Kate and Sally. 'I'll send it to my parents.' He stood between the two women. They grinned; he did not. His half-smile is inscrutable. It turned out to be my favourite photograph of Drew. There is no sign of his recent illness. He is looking straight into the camera, straight at me. It is a look of love — and I was a complete shit. It was thanks to Drew that I was on this ship, but I had

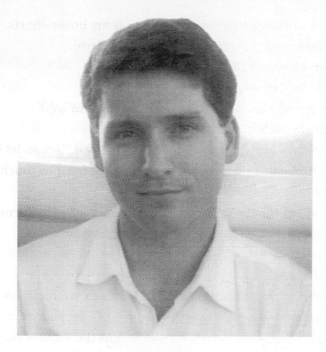

Drew on the bridge of the Sky Princess.

repaid his kindness with betrayal. Did he suspect what I had done?

Why had I seduced Chip? Boredom, loneliness, fear of commitment? A last fling before settling down with Drew? Nothing had happened in the same way that nothing had happened between Drew and the boy in Nice. Revenge never entered my mind. The non-affair was more like a wilful attempt to jeopardise my future happiness with Drew. It was as if knowing I could finally have what I wanted made me no longer want it. Or did I?

My behaviour disgusted me. I was no stranger to self-loathing yet I still considered myself a fundamentally decent person. However, this was not the only time that I had acted in a despicable manner. I had once betrayed Alex to Robert. It was while they were going through their protracted, messy break-up. My loyalties lay with Alex yet Robert kept coming to me for support. Eventually, tired of being torn in two, jealous and angry at the way Alex seemed to be squandering everything I hankered for – a long-term relationship with a handsome young man – I told Robert about Alex's pathological promiscuity. He had frequently been unfaithful to his lover in all of the nine years they had been together. I naïvely hoped that Robert would simply swap Alex for me – he had suggested such a course of action on more than one occasion – but, of course, he did not. He went home and confronted Alex with what I had told him. Then Alex told me what Robert had done. Our friendship survived; their relationship died.

My shame at betraying Alex had not stopped me betraying Drew. If my so-called general goodness depended on not having the opportunity to behave badly, then that was not goodness at all. I was as weak as everybody else. It was easy to be well-behaved when you were alone.

After the tour of the bridge Kate and Sally went off to prepare themselves for the gala night dinner. They only had three hours. Drew and I had a cocktail and watched the sun sink into the sea. Back in the cabin we had sex in the shower.

Somehow it felt different. Better. Something had changed. As soon as the Parade of the Baked Alaska was over we returned to our room, stripped off our penguin suits, and showered again. We were no longer just having sex: we were making love.

On the final night of the cruise Drew produced a bottle of Krug from his case. Neither of us had tasted it before. At midnight we went for a walk on the top deck. A million stars, a warm breeze and not a soul to be seen. The hissing, phosphorescent wake unfurled behind us. We held hands. We kissed. It was ridiculously romantic, a moment of pure corn. It was great.

4

BAD IDEAS

We parted at Victoria Station. Drew went off to Paddington and I took a cab back to the flat. It felt odd for us to be going in opposite directions. Our public farewell was low-key, undemonstrative, frustratingly inappropriate. The trip had made us closer.

I was afraid that our new-found intimacy would cool once we were back in Britain's bleak midwinter. However, the cruise, in spite of everything, had been a romantic holiday, not a holiday romance. An unexpected honeymoon. It had proved that I was meant to be part of a twosome. I missed Drew. It felt odd eating alone, going to bed alone, having no one to talk to. Drew, without me even realising it, had become an integral, essential, part of my life – and I hoped I could spend the rest of it with him. We made a good double act. Two days later, when he came to stay for the weekend, our first embrace gave me a rush greater than any experienced at the gym. Being with him made me feel whole again. I knew then that Drew was the man for me. This sudden knowledge made me bashful; Drew sensed the change in me and smiled. We hugged once more. My joy was mixed with utter relief. The search for Mr Right was finally over.

The following day *The Mystery of Morse* was broadcast on ITV. I heard my voice just once – asking John Thaw 'why?' in the trailer he used while working on location – and saw my name listed in the credits as 'Consultant'. Better still, my book was advertised after the documentary. That would boost sales. Things were starting to move.

On 20 January Bill Clinton was inaugurated as the 42nd President of the United States. However, a far more momentous event took place that evening: the 'last' episode of *Inspector Morse* went out. Almost 19 million people saw me sitting next to Thaw during the title sequence. I was actually nervous until I disappeared from view. My article about being an extra in 'Twilight of the Gods' had appeared that morning along with an incriminating photograph. I was pathetically proud even though I looked like Oscar Wilde. It was not every day you saw yourself in the *Mirror*. Normally I did not like the way I looked. I was not alone – one of the film crew, powdering my shiny nose yet again, had fondly remarked: 'You can't polish shit.'

However, five months had passed since then, and I no longer resembled the portly Irish playwright. The two curls on either side of my forehead disappeared as my hair grew longer. My cheekbones gradually reappeared as I worked off my chubbiness at the gym. I was maintaining my exercise regime, sweating away to Stakka Bo's 'Here We Go Again', even though it still felt as unlikely as a Swedish rap group. The holiday and the flu had each taken their toll. Straining against the now-familiar Nautilus equipment gave a new meaning to being back in harness.

I had wanted long hair ever since my father insisted on my having a short-back-and-sides throughout the shaggy 1970s. At the start of every term classmates and teachers would ritually tease me. There was nothing I could do. I was following in my father's footsteps – he had been to Lancaster Royal Grammar School as well – and had to take his lead in fashion too. At least I was allowed to wear flares at home. Now, though, I could please myself and required a new look to match my new life.

'You're looking good,' said Alex. 'I would never have guessed it but having longer hair suits you. So does the tan. Even the fact that you're going to a gym is beginning to show. You don't stoop so much. You know, I could almost fancy you. Well, if I was really desperate.'

I was surprised rather than flattered. Alex rarely gave compliments, even back-handed ones. 'What do you want?'

'Nothing. Just speaking my mind as usual. Leaving *Time Out* was a good move. You've been much happier and calmer since you got out of that place.'

I did not dare tell him that I wanted to return to the fold. A plum job was coming up in the film section. It would be fun to work with Geoff again. Freelance life was full of variety but it had turned out to be precarious too. The security of a staff job was becoming ever more tempting: Tower House, where *Time Out* was based in Covent Garden, still felt like home even if it was crumbling and cramped. The football pitch-sized offices of national newspapers were daunting in comparison. Serried ranks of heads staring at computer screens and muttering into phones: battery farms for journalists. Full appreciation of something often only comes with its loss.

Nevertheless, there was no going back. The management regarded me as a traitor. Still, Alex was not the only person who saw me in a different light. I seemed to be attracting more glances in the street. Of course, they could have been thinking 'what the hell was that?', but somehow I did not think so. Perhaps they recognised me from *Inspector Morse* or the *Mirror*.

'Yeah, right,' said Alex. 'Mark Sanderson, international superstar! Dream on. It's nothing to do with that. I told you it was no good just sitting at home, moping and hoping, a bitter old queen. You finally got off your flabby arse and made something happen. You've started to regain your self-respect. If you like yourself then other people will too.' He sighed. 'If you keep going you might even have a body like mine one day . . . Well, perhaps not.'

As far as I was concerned Drew deserved as much credit as I did for the new me. Love is good for self-esteem. On

Australia Day, 26 January, he sent me a list of all the things we had done since our first meeting. We had been through a lot together in four months. On Valentine's Day I received eight cards. Each one had a letter inscribed inside the front. When read in the correct order they spelled out I LOVE YOU. The year before I had not received a single card. Hardly a week went by without some sort of billet-doux arriving from Drew. Once I got an apparently meaningless mass of colourful letters snipped from magazines and sealed between two sheets of clear sticky-backed plastic – an accompanying note told me to use 'this specially punched piece of paper as a cipher-key'. The cut-outs in the blank sheet revealed MARK, I LOVE YOU; DREW. Every month a card celebrated our latest 'anniversary'.

We were a happy couple if the world left us alone but, of course, it did not. Drew needed to find a new job and I needed a new home. The couple who had been burgled upstairs had split up, gone their separate ways, and let out the flat to three students who did not go to bed before 1.30am. The clomping across the ceiling drove me mad. Water started to seep across it when they used the washing machine. When they showered, soapy water cascaded down the walls of my bathroom. Complaining to them, their land-lords and the letting agency made little difference. I had to get out.

At the end of February Drew was offered a job in Kuwait. It paid £1,000 a week, plus bonuses, and came with free accommodation and a car. I did not want him to take it. We were apart too much as it was. A friend offered me a three-month contract as a television researcher at his production company. It paid £400 a week. I accepted it. In the meantime, though, I had to go to Finland. The PR company had liked my work on *The Snapper* and offered me the same brief on a film called *The Big Freeze*. I gave Drew a set of keys to Shakespeare Walk. 'They're yours to keep.' I had never given my keys to anyone before. I trusted him implicitly. Besides, I needed someone to keep an eye on the leaks.

Film crews are like close-knit families: they do not like strangers in their midst. They and the cast have to work as a team, usually away from home, so an us-and-them mentality often develops. Myriad things can go wrong while shooting on location, and spectators only make matters worse. As a journalist I had learned that the best method of getting a story on set was to keep quiet and keep out of the way. You kept your eyes and ears open and your mouth closed. A good producer would ensure that you got to talk to the right people eventually. However, you had to be patient.

My hotel room, like the rest of the establishment, was spotlessly clean, well-appointed and utterly anonymous. After checking in I succeeded in tracking down one of the co-producers. He was preparing a party in the hotel kitchens. The shoot was almost over. However, no one seemed in a mood to celebrate. The English crew sat at two tables, the Finns at another. Eric Sykes, the director, ate with his producers. His co-stars – Bob Hoskins, Donald Pleasence, Sir John Mills and his wife – dined at another. I needed to interview all of them, but not tonight. I left them alone, concentrated on the Australian chardonnay, and slowly got drunk. It was a real pleasure to know, as I slumped into bed, there were no hyperactive tenants above my head.

The next day a minibus finally arrived to take me to the set: a summer-house twenty-five kilometres outside Tampere. The sun shone on snow, ice and fir tree. There was nothing else to see. The large, wooden house, simply but superbly designed, would have seemed familiar to any devotee of Ingmar Bergman. In *The Big Freeze* it was being used as a home for retired actors. Tiptoeing over snaking cables, I made my way through a maze of stainless steel cases. Donald Pleasence sat on a chair in the middle of the room. He was slurping soup as water trickled on to his head. I thought I had left the leaks at home.

The Big Freeze was a silent comedy in the same vein as *The Plank*. In that film Eric Sykes had co-starred with Tommy Cooper. This time his partner was Bob Hoskins. They played a father-and-son team of bumbling plumbers. Hoskins said he was 'flabbergasted' to have been invited to fill the boots of the late, great Cooper. 'It was like Stan Laurel asking you to take the place of Oliver Hardy,' he told me when I cornered him in his caravan after lunch. 'The film is about two totally stupid people who are the last people on earth to consider themselves funny – and that's what is funny.' Acting was a deadly serious business to Hoskins. I had been a fan of his ever since *The Long Good Friday*. He had not lost his talent for Cockney menace. I would have liked to talk to him about his other films but my job was to produce kind words for a press release, not a revealing, in-depth interview. Thirty minutes was all I needed and all I got.

Donald Pleasence was in a more expansive mood. He was treating a bout of bronchitis with regular doses of cheap wine poured from a magnum. It was good practice for his role as the noisy eater. 'My soup-slurping is heard throughout the film,' he said. 'It irritates the other inhabitants of the home. I like to do comedy but I don't get much chance nowadays. I used to do nothing else.' He assumed a vacant expression. It was extraordinary how he could make his baldness comical. He was famous for playing sinister characters such as Blofeld, the Persian-petting head of SPECTRE, in *You Only Live Twice*. Then again, he had appeared in over 200 movies. Why did he keep on working? 'Wives are very expensive. You'll find out one day. I've no doubt that I have made too many films but I shall go on working until I can't do it any more. That is to say, until I can't stand up, I can't remember the lines or become ill. I don't see any sense in retiring because there's nothing else I want to do full-time.'

Both men were lucky to be doing something they loved, something they were good at – and getting paid handsomely for it to boot. That was one definition of success, a key to happiness. Drew was well-paid in computing but would rather have been teaching young children; I loved writing but did not earn enough. Pots of money or personal fulfilment: it was a frustrating choice. Nevertheless, I now knew having a lover made life more bearable. It was all a question of compromise and consolation.

I hung around for the rest of the afternoon but failed to bag any more interviews. Waiting often proved to be the hardest part of the job. Night fell. I cadged a ride back to the hotel with the Finnish co-producer, had a swim in the chilly, indoor pool then ventured into the sauna.

A seven-a-side football team wandered about in the nude drinking a beer called Koff. They were young, blond and beautiful, totally at ease with themselves and their mates. There was none of the atmosphere of subtle tension which pervades British locker rooms. English men lowered their heads as soon as anyone lowered their trousers, as if it were a crime to see another man's body. If they were not cringingly self-conscious they were aggressively exhibitionist, both attitudes indicative of unease. I watched the boys with more admiration than lust. I had never looked like that and never would. The fact that I was in this room at all, and pretty relaxed as well, was remarkable in itself. Now I felt lucky too. I had come a long way in six months. That loser lurking by the lake in France was no longer me.

There was a message waiting for me when I returned to my room. It was from Drew.

'Hello, Possum. What's up?'

'Your mother called half an hour ago. She was shocked when you didn't answer. I explained that I was house-sitting for you but she didn't sound too convinced. I keep expecting the police to arrive. You better call her.'

'Okay. I'll call you back when I've spoken to her.'

My mother did not know that I was in Finland. I had told

my father but he had forgotten to mention it. I called my parents once a week without fail. It was one of my weekend chores. It felt like a chore because there was so much I could not talk to them about. The reticence was more for their sake than mine. It was as if they needed protecting from the real me. I did not want to be a disappointment. My father regularly asked me when I was going to get 'a proper job' – and he did not know the half of it. For instance, the fact that his son was gay. The sight of two footballers kissing would provoke a rant about the evils of homosexuality: 'I'm going to leave the country before it's made compulsory.' I always spoke to both my parents but did not like repeating myself. I relied on each of them to relay the gist of their conversation to the other. Suggestions that they invest in a speakerphone were ignored.

'It's me. You haven't called the police, have you?'

'No, but I thought about it.'

'Why? A burglar wouldn't answer the phone. If it rang he'd just rip it out.'

'You never know these days.'

'Did Drew sound like a burglar?'

'I suppose he was rather polite. He's not British, is he?'

'He's from Australia. His dad's a dentist too.'

'Oh, well, there's no harm done. I was just surprised not to hear your voice.'

'Dad should have told you I was away. I'd still have called you on Sunday as usual. There's not much to do here. I saw John Mills going for a walk in the snow this morning. He was wearing pink moon-boots.' And I was off, creating a verbal smokescreen, veering away from what was most important. I would have loved to have said, *should* have said: 'Actually, Mum, Drew is my boyfriend. We've been seeing each other for six months now and I like him a lot.' But I did not. My mother never spoke to Drew again.

I had been told there was no point going out to the summer-house again because everyone had a full schedule. Mr Sykes would talk to me back in England when the filming was over. My interview with John Mills was postponed several times. In the end I was invited up to his suite at 8.30 on Sunday evening.

He gave an immaculate performance as he sat on the sofa with his wife. The remains of their dinner were still on the coffee table in front of them. The scene in the suite was one of organised chaos.

'I had a telephone call from a gentleman called Eric Sykes just two weeks ago,' said Sir John. 'He said, "I'd like you to do something." I said, "What?" He said, "I'd like you to come and act in a picture with me in Finland. Are you working?" I said, "Strangely enough, no. What's the picture called?" and he said, "*The Big Freeze*." I said, "What's my part like?" He said, "Very funny." I said, "Give me an idea." "It's quite simple," he said. "You poke me in the stomach with an umbrella." Well, of course I told him it's the one part I've always wanted to play.'

The role of The Well-Dressed Man required Sir John to play himself. The debonair old trouper was continually being recognised by Bob Hoskins' plumber who, having seen *Ryan's Daughter*, would point at Sir John and pull a face. 'I was fond of Michael in *Ryan's Daughter* because I got the Oscar for it,' said Sir John. 'I've always liked awards and prizes. However, of all my screen roles the one that gives me least pain is Willie Mossop in *Hobson's Choice*. For sheer pleasure I've always gone for Willie.'

It was time to turn off the tape-recorder. The affection and respect the Millses had for each other was obvious. No wonder their marriage had lasted for decades. I wondered if Drew and I would still be together when we were in our eighties.

The following week I started work at Panoptic Productions. I was to be the researcher on two documentaries that would form part of a series on Channel 4 called *Bad Ideas of the Twentieth Century*. The first, 'Youthism', would be presented by Germaine Greer, the feminist writer, and shot in England. The second, 'Bodyism', would be presented by Erica Jong, the American novelist, and shot in New York.

The firm was based in Heddon Street, a cul-de-sac off Regent Street. Its office essentially comprised one big attic space. Three boxed-off cubicles under the eaves provided each of the company directors – Jean, Michael and Christine – with rooms of their own. The rest of the loft was taken up with six desks, two black leather sofas and a kitchenette. Gerard, the baby of this dysfunctional family, lived in a tiny edit suite by the front door. The roost was ruled by Mad Mary from Sydney, Nova Scotia. She had been an assistant editor on Julien Temple's *Absolute Beginners* but, for some reason, now found being Michael's PA far more fun.

I soon discovered why. Every evening at half-past six, cries of 'sun's over the yard-arm!' would come from at least one of the cubicles. Mary would scuttle to the fridge and, within seconds, a bottle of champagne would pop its cork. It was an excellent way to end the day, a reward for all the hours spent on the telephone trying to find a telegenic Pakistani family in Bradford or a war memorial in a picturesque location. The dead soldier on the worktop would soon be joined by another – and another. The Panoptic gang were my kind of people. I dubbed them The Heddonists.

Drew, unsurprisingly, resented my coming home late and drunk. His contract with WHSmith in Swindon had ended, so he came to stay with me. He would do the laundry and the shopping, and there would often be fresh flowers awaiting my return, yet there was no getting away from the fact that the flat was too small. Although we retired to separate rooms each night, neither of us was getting enough sleep. Loud music from upstairs disturbed Drew in the living room; heavy feet woke me in the bedroom. The leaks had at last been sealed but the noise levels were just the same.

The lack of a job affected Drew more than the lack of sleep: he, at least, could snooze through the afternoon if he wished. He must have been lonely, stuck in Stoke Newington all day, waiting for me to come home. The Kuwaiti offer was still on the table.

'The money is very good.' Drew had been in a sulk ever since I had got in. Eight o'clock was not that late. I could not start making calls to New York until 3pm.

'True, but what would you spend it on? There's nothing to do over there.'

'There's nothing to do over here.'

'That's not my fault. I can't have lunch with you every day.' At the end of my first week at Panoptic we had rendezvoused at the café in Beak Street where we had gone on the day we first met. It was only a minute from the office.

'I know that, but it's not much fun being here by myself – especially with the animals upstairs.'

'Why don't you go and check on your flat in Oxford?'

He looked at me. 'I let it go.'

'Why? Where's all your stuff?'

'It was a waste of money. I don't need to live in Oxford now I'm not working in Swindon. My stuff's in storage in King's Cross.'

'I can't believe you didn't tell me. I said you could come to stay, not move in.'

'Exactly. I was afraid you'd say no if I asked.' He buried his face in my chest. 'I can easily find another place.'

'Drew, I'm not going to kick you out. I gave you my keys, didn't I? What if your next job is in Oxford? You had a nice place there.'

'Apart from the prowler.'

'Did you ever see anyone?'

'Someone knocked on the window once.'

'Who?'

'I don't know. It was dark. I was in bed. It made me jump.'

I gave him a hug. 'Well, you're safe now. You're with me. You can always ask me anything, you know. Anything. I would have said yes.' I sounded certain now, but I was not sure how I would have reacted had I not been faced with a *fait accompli.*

A full-time job made it difficult for me to stick to my exercise routine. I had to go to the gym in the evening and at week-ends, when it was busier. I hated it when someone, reeking of oniony sweat, stood beside you, their blank face failing to mask their impatience as they waited to use a particular piece of equipment.

Spring finally arrived. When Drew disappeared for a few days to show an Australian friend round England I was sur-prised how much I missed him. A card arrived with an eye, a heart and a U on the front: 'Mark, wherever in the world we are, whatever we are doing, whether employed or unem-ployed, whether freelance or not, I will love you. Drew xxx.'

It seemed like a good idea at the time: a weekend on board a canal barge with Alex and Johnny, his new boyfriend. 'Oh, do come. It'll be so boring without you.' I knew Alex and knew about canals. I had done a project about them when I was at junior school. Alex was afraid that he would have to do all the hard graft. However, the prospect of two nights of uninter-rupted sleep was too tempting to refuse.

I took the Friday off work. Alex and Johnny collected

Drew and I and then drove to Gayton in Northamptonshire. We were given a tour of the 65-foot barge and shown how to operate it. Johnny, a capable ex-public schoolboy, took the helm. He had done this before. The owner came with us to ensure that we knew what we were doing, then hopped on his bike and cycled back along the towpath. We were on our own.

The *Stonechat* chugged along. Drew sat in the bow with his camcorder. The rest of us stood in the stern admiring the scenery. It was early April but most of the trees, apart from a few flowering cherries, were still bare. The white blossom seemed incongruously festive. We negotiated Blisworth Tunnel, the longest navigable tunnel in Britain, without mishap and, full of enthusiasm, ascended a flight of seven locks.

We moored at dusk near Grafton Regis. The silence was blissful. We opened a bottle of champagne and watched the orange sun sink behind a distant, hill-top church. The barge was surprisingly comfortable. Its kitchen was modern and equipped with a full range of appliances. After dinner, courtesy of Marks & Spencer, we played strip Trivial Pursuit. I was the only one to keep my trousers on. Johnny ended up doing press-ups in the nude.

There were three beds on board, all small doubles. Alex and Johnny had the one at the front, Drew had the one at the back. I helped him convert it from the table we had all just been sitting round and got into it with him. Half an hour later I went to my own bed in the middle. I slept like a log.

*

We shared our breakfast with some greedy ducks then set off through the mist to Cosgrove. We stocked up with drinking water, went through a single lock, and found ourselves thirty-five feet up in the air. The Ouse Aqueduct crossed the river which formed the boundary between Northamptonshire and Buckinghamshire. The ancient engineering was more impressive than the view.

We puttered past railway works and brickworks, empty fields and drowned sheep. The speed limit on the Grand Union Canal was 4mph, frustratingly slow. It was illegal to make a wash. Alex, however, soon became bored and mysteriously lost the ability to steer. He zigzagged between the sides and spread mayhem down below as he repeatedly rammed into the bank. Captain Johnny took over the rudder. Alex, giggling hysterically, retreated to the kitchen. He had got what he wanted.

The fact that you had to turn the rudder in the opposite direction to the way you wished to go seemed illogical. Drew, who loved boats, succeeded only in sending the barge into the middle of a large hawthorn thicket. He should have slowed down but accelerated instead: the brass handle of the rudder, hooked round a branch, bent upwards from 45 to 70 degrees. It looked like a rocket launcher and thereafter provoked several wry comments from passers-by. I smiled thinly and stared straight ahead.

It started to rain after lunch and did not let up for the rest of the day. Alex and Drew stayed inside reading newspapers or watching television. Johnny and I took it in turns at the helm. Golden-haired and affectionate, he was a human Labrador, far too nice for Alex. He was besotted with my friend and, not unintelligent, already afraid of losing him. I knew that he would, but said nothing. Alex was going through a toyboy phase. It was too soon after his break-up with Robert for him to settle down with anyone else. I could see that Drew liked Johnny and sympathised with his plight. However, he had a mental block about his name and kept calling him John only to realise his mistake almost immediately so that it came out sounding like 'John-E'. Alex thought Drew was doing this on purpose. The atmosphere became tense. Any conversation degenerated into bickering and bitching. I maintained my position at the rudder. Water trickled down the back of my neck. When we passed a housing estate it started raining stones as well.

We moored on the outskirts of Milton Keynes. Everyone felt in need of a drink. We ate after *Blind Date* then played Pictionary. At 10.30 we went to bed. It had been a bad day. Drew broke down in my arms. He told me how much he needed me.

'You become a different person when you're with Alex. Harder. He brings out the worst in you.'

'He's my best friend. We've been through a lot together. You'll like him more when you get to know him better. He puts on a front like the rest of us.'

'I don't.'

'No. I don't suppose you do. That's one of the reasons I like you. Drew, I love you. I'm not going to leave you. You'll get another job soon. We all go through bad patches. As soon as I sell Shakespeare Walk we'll be able to make a new start together. You have to trust me.'

The next morning we retraced our route back to Gayton. None of us wanted to open or close a lock-gate ever again. Alex was relieved to be behind the wheel of his VW Golf. He said he was safer on dry land. We hurtled down the M1 back to London.

Drew was offered a job at Thames Water in Reading. It paid £1,000 a week. He accepted it. He started work on St George's Day and Shakespeare's birthday: 23 April was an auspicious date. At 5pm that evening he called me from his bed and breakfast: 'I can't stay here.' I did not point out how close Oxford was to Reading, I just did my best to reassure him. The conversation ended when Drew said, 'Let's get a place together.' I called the estate agents immediately. If I could not sell Shakespeare Walk I would let it. When I was still awake at 3am, staring into the dark as drunken children jumped around upstairs, I knew we had made the right decision. Later that morning, before I went to the gym, I got their telephone number from directory enquiries and did not hang up until someone answered. Five minutes later I did it again. And again.

There was a postcard waiting for me when I got home. A cartoon koala bear sat at a typewriter: 'MISS YOU MISS YOU MISS YOU . . . MORE THAN I CAN SAY'. It was from Drew. 'I'm sitting on a strange bed in a strange town and my mind keeps wandering back to thoughts of you. I want so desperately to be with you and the time when we are next together cannot come soon enough. I hope you feel the same.' I did.

Half an hour later the whole house shook as a huge IRA bomb exploded in the City, killing one person and injuring dozens of others. When the sofa beneath you suddenly shakes, the fact that death can happen at any moment is brought home to you. I had always had a fatalistic attitude towards terrorism. There were many reasons to avoid Oxford Street but the possibility that a litter-bin might explode as you walked past was not one of them. Now, though, I had someone else to worry about. I was relieved that Drew was out of London and therefore, relatively speaking, out of harm's way. I already knew that I would do anything to protect him.

5

TOO GOOD TO BE TRUE

We moved into Packington Street on Saturday 15 May. The upper maisonette was easily the best flat we had seen. The one above a shop in Cross Street had been too shabby; the one in St Paul Street too cramped. There was a living room and kitchen on the first floor, two bedrooms and a bathroom on the second floor. We had our own front door on the ground floor and, on the first floor, our own back door too. It opened on to a roof terrace from where a long spiral staircase led down into the garden. This patch of jungle was Drew's favourite feature. He had missed not having any outdoor space. I loved my little bedroom. I was quite content to let Drew have the large one at the front: it was too noisy for me. The fact that there would be no one above or directly below me when I went to bed filled me with utter relief.

The house was in a Victorian terrace of white stucco-fronted properties that stretched all the way from Essex Road to Prebend Street. It had been converted into two architect-designed flats in 1990 but the upper one had remained unoccupied ever since. I liked the idea that no one had lived here before: we were making a new start in a new home. Its high ceilings and large sash windows made it light and airy but such a des res was by no means cheap to rent. It cost £910 per month. 'We can afford it,' said Drew. 'We're both working again.'

I had wanted to live in Islington for years. Now, thanks to Drew, I could finally knock the six off my postcode. We were in the heart of N1. Islington Green and Camden Passage were just around the corner, the Angel a five-minute walk away. I had been past the end of Packington Street countless times on the Number 73 bus but, until the estate agent turned off Essex Road, had never been down it. You could see St Mary's Church on Upper Street from the terrace, St James's on Prebend Street from the kitchen and St John the Evangelist's in Duncan Terrace from the living room. We were at the centre of a sacred triangle. It was a charmed location. We were safe at last.

It did not take long to load up the removals van. I was allowed to ride in the cab to Packington Street. When I said I had been driven out of Shakespeare Walk by noisy neighbours the driver told me that it was a good thing I had not lived in the next street, as Milton Grove was known for its poltergeists. They were very active during the 1960s, apparently. After almost six years I was both sad and glad to be going.

Drew arrived from Reading early in the afternoon. Hot and dusty from unpacking, I came down to meet him in the hall. We kissed for the first time in the house. An hour later Howard and Sarah turned up. My old schoolfriend helped me construct the single bed I had bought in John Lewis the week before and tack a blanket over the window. There were no curtain rails. The boiler had seized up from lack of use. We called a plumber.

That evening we warmed the flat with chilled champagne, ordered pizza and watched the Republic of Ireland win the Eurovision Song Contest again. Drew was appalled by our ruthless British patriotism, not our lack of musical taste. I soon realised that Drew had probably wanted us to spend our first evening in Packington Street alone, but I felt in need of some neutral moral support. Setting up home together was a big step. I was nervous. I had lived with Alex in Manchester, I had once shared a flat with Howard in Bethnal Green, but I had never lived with a lover. It could all go horribly wrong. I suppose he felt the same way too. We made up in the kitchen when Howard and Sarah left in a taxi then made out amid the chaos of his room. It was a real novelty to go upstairs to bed. Afterwards we lay in each other's arms and listened to the silence.

On the following Monday I saw Howard again. It was the first day of the 'Youthism' shoot so we had all gone back to school. Germaine Greer wanted to canvass some young people on their views about getting old. Howard taught

classics at University College School in Hampstead, so I persuaded him to get us permission to do some filming there.
Germaine began by writing '*Tempus edax rerum*' on the black-
board: 'time eats all things.' The articulate teenagers were
captivated by her outspokenness and, although she was old
enough to be their mother, responded to her flirting. She had
even put on her own version of school uniform – grey skirt,
blue blouse, striped tie – for the occasion.

Afterwards Michael, the producer, Lenny, the director,
and I took her for a drink in a wine bar on Haverstock Hill.
We had been awestruck when we first met Germaine in her
rooms at Newnham College, Cambridge. The superstar aca-
demic proceeded to give us a tutorial. She had a clear idea of
how she wanted to illustrate her thesis that worshipping youth
was a Very Bad Thing but had no desire to discuss practical
matters like budgets and permissions. That, after all, was our
job. She was the celebrity; we were her entourage. I liked her
immediately. She had brains and beauty, and had been playing
the fame game a long time. One morning, in bed with
Warren Beatty, she had seen herself on breakfast television.
Beatty immediately got up and got dressed. He did not sleep
with chicks who were more famous than him.

The collaborative nature of working in television presented
new challenges. Putting pictures to other people's words,
illustrating their ideas, is not as rewarding as expressing your
own, and it is not something that you can do by yourself.
The kindness of strangers was essential. Journalism is all

about telling the truth; being a researcher seemed mainly to involve telling lics. The job was to get the right people in the right place at the right time. If the director wanted a young man and an old woman to run an assault course then you had to find your victims, get permission to film at the police training centre in Hendon, take out special insurance, and make sure the nervous athletes got to the location in time. This required countless pleading telephone calls and lots of little white lies. In the end it was quicker to forget about the truth and tell the person what they wanted to hear.

Television gobbles up real life to produce a fleeting facsimile of it. The medium consumes the lives of those who work in it too – the distinction between professional and private life disappears. One's friends, family and acquaintances are all fair game, there to be exploited if the production demands it. Howard was happy to receive a bottle of champagne for his help but Jason, the young man who had given me a fitness test at the N16 gym and who agreed to take part in 'Youthism', did not drink. He even found me a grey-haired grandmother fit enough to be his competitor on the assault course. The two of them spent an afternoon swinging on ropes and clambering over obstacles. They were the director's playthings and earned every penny of their pittance. Three months later, after several enquiries about when he was going to be on TV, I had to tell Jason that the sequence had not made it into the final programme.

Writing was so much simpler. When I sat at my desk at home I did not need to obtain anyone's permission or have to rely on someone's goodwill. It was just me and the computer. All the running around was done in my head. I was in control.

I had wanted to be a writer for as long as I could remember. On my seventh birthday my parents gave me a desk. I asked what was under the dust-sheet as soon as I ran into their bedroom. 'Just a big pile of old books,' said my father. 'Have a look if you don't believe me . . .' I was even more delighted when I lifted up the sloping lid and found the desk filled with presents. There were more presents in the seat of the chair underneath it as well. I filled page after page of my school exercise book describing what I had done in the holidays. There was always so much to say. I liked trying to turn the world into words.

Islington had long been a haunt of writers. George Orwell had lived in Canonbury Square. Today, it seemed you could not go into Marks & Spencer without seeing Adam Mars-Jones in his biking leathers or Penelope Lively loading her yellow and black checked bag. Nick, with whom I stayed at Le Lac, had lived here with his first wife, Janet Hobhouse, the American novelist. Once upon a time Charles Lamb had lived in Duncan Terrace. Now Peter Ackroyd lived there, as did Douglas Adams. Drew was a huge fan of *The Hitch-Hiker's Guide to the Galaxy* and could not believe he now lived in the very same neighbourhood as its author. Hugo Williams, the poet, lived round the corner in Raleigh Street and, a couple of streets away, back in 1967, Kenneth Halliwell, before killing himself, had bashed in the head of Joe Orton, his lover, at the top of a house in Noel Road. It was a far cry from Cairns.

I was impressed by Drew's design for our change-of-address flyer. The collage showed a big hand coming down from the sky to raise the roof of a little house on the prairie. A Corinthian column, a spiral staircase and a giant question mark completed the picture. That about said it all. As a reward I took a detour on my way in to Panoptic and bought him a big jar of Vegemite at the Australia shop off the Strand.

'You can tell you're Australian. You nod your head when you speak.' Drew nodded. Germaine Greer was sitting on the floor of his flat. It was a surreal occasion. She had arrived in Packington Street, bedraggled and bewildered, at 9.45. The idea had been to have dinner at Granita, a modish restaurant on Upper Street, at 9pm but Germaine had got lost and we had lost the table. We were off to a club in Dalston later that evening to film careless youth having fun. As Drew and I lived nearby it had seemed to make sense to rendezvous here. The crew would make their own way to Hackney.

Mad Mary plied Germaine with champagne while I went into the kitchen to raid the fridge. We had not been expecting guests. 'Let's have a carpet picnic,' said Drew. He helped me carry the bread, cheese, salad and houmous into the living room. Everyone sat on the floor. The sofa-bed and two director's chairs, the only pieces of furniture, looked lost on the sea of grey carpet. We had been in Packington Street for just a fortnight. Floor-to-ceiling bookshelves now filled the alcoves either side of the chimney breast. Ian, the carpenter, had also fitted the curtain rails but nothing hung from them yet. The windows in my old place had shutters. I had spent a satisfying morning arranging my books on the new shelves, which had cost me a whole week's wages. Walter Abish was eight storeys above Zinovy Zinik. Anthony Powell was right: books did furnish a room.

The library was my pride and joy. It had grown as I had grown. It represented countless Christmas presents and birthday presents, hard-earned pocket-money investments, relics of my university reading list and years of combing second-hand book stalls and bookshops. I had always worked with books. My first job had been in the mail-room of a literary agency, my second was writing blurbs for Jonathan Cape, the publisher. Even when I was at *Time Out* I regularly reviewed books for the magazine. Now I reviewed them for the *Independent on Sunday* and was trying to write another one of my own. A proper one this time, a novel. I loved books. They were more reliable than people.

The club was called Labrynth. Its owners may not have been familiar with Greek mythology – or a dictionary – but they knew that any mention of drugs in connection with the place would spell disaster. I had to promise that Ecstasy would not be a topic of conversation. Germaine interviewed a music journalist outside the dive in Dalston Lane. The shuffling queue, apart from one lantern-jawed clubber, pretended to ignore the camera. 'Listen to the guy,' the boy told her. 'You know fuck-all.'

I was Germaine's walker for the evening. We arrived in a cloudburst. Exhaust fumes and fast-food smells filled the humid air. I put my arm round Germaine's waist and, holding a golf umbrella aloft, guided her through the crowds. Drew, Mary and the crew followed on behind.

We descended into an inner circle of hell. Noise, heat and smoke crashed over us. A sea of young bodies, arms raised, swayed to the music, a giant anemone feeding in the gloom. The umbrella came in useful as we forced our way through the waves of glistening dancers and upstairs to the VIP suite, a grotty cubby-hole with a battered sofa and rattling fridge. Mary opened the champagne we had brought and served it in white plastic cups. Drew took some pictures. He was our stills photographer for the night. When the flash went off Germaine always managed to be smiling.

Once Lenny had got enough footage of blinking strobes and tripping teenagers we shifted to The Attic, a chill-out room at the top of the building. Germaine interviewed a bug-eyed granny who claimed to be a well-known figure on the club circuit. She was wearing bottle-green Lycra, a black bum-bag and an artificial laurel wreath on her head. Age, apparently, was all in the mind. 'I've done my best to grow old disgracefully,' said Germaine. The ancient adolescent was not convinced: 'You've got a long way to go yet.'

Mary ensured that the champagne kept flowing. It seemed to seep straight from your pores. We interlopers were the only ones drinking alcohol. Everyone else swigged from little plastic bottles of water. When the last of the vox-pops was in the can we all assembled for a group photo. Drew had no

difficulty in making us do what he wanted. It was only afterwards that I realised no one had taken a picture of him.

A minicab bounced us back to Packington Street.
Germaine refused the offer of coffee – she got straight into
her Mercedes, executed a perfect U-turn and, with the wave
of a hand, drove off into the sunrise. I seemed to be the only
one who was exhausted. All I wanted to do was sleep. Drew,
however, would not take no for an answer.

During the carpet picnic Germaine had quizzed us about our
relationship. It was quite obvious we had just moved in
together. She sympathised with the problems we faced
because Drew's visa was running out, but considered a *Green
Card*-style marriage to Mary, which she had suggested, a bad
idea. 'You may be in love now, but what about in a year's
time?'

'I have no doubts,' said Drew.

'Neither do I.' We looked at each other and smiled.

'People change,' said Germaine. 'It takes a long time to
really get to know someone. All I'm saying is that if you do go
to all that trouble, you'd better stay together.'

Her visit had made our lack of furniture painfully apparent.
The floor, in spite of the new carpet, was not that comfortable. It took six months for us to fill all the gaps. We ordered
a pair of matching sofas from a shop in Tottenham Court
Road and curtains from John Lewis. Drew successfully bid for
a wardrobe and chest of drawers in the Criterion Salerooms
on Essex Road. He would often come home on a Monday

evening to announce that he had bought something else: a couple of mirrors, a hatstand for the hall, a marble-topped table for the terrace.

Alex, who was moving from Highbury to Chiswick, sold me a wardrobe, chest of drawers, blanket box, coffee table and dining table all for £300. I was not pleased at the prospect of him living so far away. 'Well, I see a lot less of you now you're with Drew. You can always come round for tea.' I knew he was moving to be closer to his office, but I could not help thinking he was also doing it to punish me. Alex was accustomed to my being at his beck and call. If he was bored at work or depressed, he would phone me. Hearing about my life always made him feel better. It was true that I had less free time nowadays but no one could accuse me of neglect. I had been determined, right from the start, that none of my friendships should suffer because of my relationship with Drew. That was why, today, it seemed as though we always had guests. We were proud of the flat. We wanted our friends to see it – and to see that we were happy.

At the end of June my sister telephoned to say that our 74-year-old grandmother, Em, had cancer. Tests had revealed a tumour. If it proved to be malignant a kidney and her bladder might have to be removed. As far as we knew, it was the first time our family had been affected by cancer.

Our other grandparents were dead. I had always been closest to Emily, my mother's mother. She hated her name and insisted on being called Em. She had left school at fourteen

and spent most of her life working for Woolworth's. As man-
ageress of the Lancaster branch she had been able to get her
teenage grandson a part-time job stacking shelves after school
or serving on the sweet counter on Saturdays. I loathed the
grey nylon uniform but liked the £6.90 weekly wage.
However, when my grandmother retired in 1978, a malicious
junior executive moved me on to the baler.

This massive blue machine was housed in a windowless
bare-bricked room on the roof of the department store next
to the stockroom. Cardboard boxes that had held tins of sar-
dines or butter beans were fed into its maw, crushed and
eventually excreted in bales held together by plastic tape. It
was often necessary to fight one's way into the room because
it would be filled from floor to ceiling with empty boxes. A
real box room. The only way to get to the machine was to
launch yourself into the cardboard sea and flail like a drowning swimmer. Stabbed by corners, cut by edges, pricked by
staples, it was a great way to start work. The baling room was
hot, noisy and dirty. After a month I quit.

Five days after my sister's call Em was released from hospital.

'Hello, Nana. It's Mark.'

'Hello, Mark David. How are you?' She sounded just the
same.

'Never mind about me. How are you?' In the circumstances the question sounded insultingly banal.

'Not so bad. A bit tired. The tumour is malignant but my
kidneys are clear. They're not going to operate until they see
how the radiotherapy works. The consultant said there's no

immediate danger. Cancer doesn't spread very fast in old folk.'

'When will the radiotherapy start?'

'I'm waiting to hear. Maybe next month.' Sarcastic remarks would not be helpful. There was so much I wanted to say but could not. Do you blame Grandpa's cigarettes? Are you afraid? Does it hurt?

'I'll see you in three weeks. I'm coming up for Dad's birthday. Let me know if I can do anything.'

'Of course. Your mum's being very good. So what have you been up to? Found yourself a nice lady-friend yet?' She asked me this every time I called her.

'I'm too busy. I've been working on two TV documentaries. My contract ends in a couple of weeks. I want to get on with my next book.'

'Well, you know what they say about all work and no play. As long as you're happy.'

'Honestly, Nana, I've never been happier in my life.'

I wanted to tell her about Drew. She would have probably taken the news better than my parents. She had already given up dropping hints about great-grandchildren. However, she had enough to deal with at the moment. Besides, such revelations should be made in person, not on the telephone.

I replaced the receiver. Drew was lying on the sofa-bed. The new sofas were not due until August. 'Okay?'

'Yes.' I burst into tears. It surprised us both. He came and put his arms around me.

*

The virtual-reality sex-suit was ready to take to New York but it would not be going in my suitcase. Camille Paglia, the outspoken feminist critic; Dr Maynard, a specialist in eating disorders; and Lypsinka, a notable drag queen, were all lined up to talk to Erica Jong: there was no need, and no money, for me to go to America. The budget for 'Bodyism' had been stretched too far. I was not disappointed. A couple of nights at a health spa – where towel-clad Erica would sweat the answers out of some female dicters in the steam room – would have been fun but I did not want to be separated from Drew.

Michael and Lenny returned from the Big Apple bearing gifts. Lenny gave me a pair of handcuffs – 'for you and Drew' – that looked real but were not. He would not let me forget our recce to an S&M dungeon in West Brompton. The windowless bedroom in Cathcart Road was lined with rubber, draped with chains and packed with mysterious gadgets. Its buxom bottle-blonde owner, just about wearing a black leather bustier, had taken exception to my flippant remarks. My blood ran cold when she said, playing with a nipple clamp, 'I'm going to have to do something about you.'

The wrap party to celebrate the completion of filming – and the end of my contract – was held in the Panoptic office on 13 July. Drew was in bed when I got back at 1.30am. He was still in bed when I got up seven hours later: 'I've got tummy ache.' I sent him to see a doctor at the local practice where I had just registered. A gastric virus was diagnosed; starvation and sugary drinks prescribed.

I spent the day nursing Drew and my hangover. He had

been working too hard lately. He rose at 5.45am each day to go to Reading and it was often after 9pm before he got home. Even then he would sometimes have to talk a colleague through a difficult procedure on the telephone. The conversation could last five minutes or an hour. Either way, said Drew, 'that's another £80 in the bank'. It did not matter if it was a weekend or the middle of the night: if the Thames Water computer system needed attention then Drew was paid to give it. We were grateful for the overtime. Credit-card spending sprees created mounting interest fees.

I read James Ellroy's *The Big Nowhere* on the train to Lancaster. I had not been home since Christmas. I was glad to get out of London but wished Drew were with me. It would have been fun showing the former teacher round my old school. My parents lived on Cannon Hill, where Cromwell's forces were supposed to have gathered to attack the castle. They had bought the house in 1978 when they had moved from Chester to be closer to their own ageing parents. This meant I could stop boarding at Lancaster Royal Grammar School and become a day-boy — or, as the boarders said with mindless inevitability, a 'gay-boy'. As I trudged up the hill from the station I was following in the footsteps of my younger self. I had lugged my Adidas bag of text-books up the steep incline on countless rainy afternoons. The road was so narrow it was impossible to avoid the spray from passing cars. Later, as a sixth-former, returning from a midnight screening of a film at the Duke's Playhouse, I would walk up the badly-lit hill

expecting at any moment someone to jump out of the rho-
dodendron bushes that protected the sprawling Edwardian
villas from prying eyes. Years later someone ambushed my
father in exactly this way. The mugger fled empty-handed.

As you reached the brow of the hill, breathing deeply, the
hulk of the nuclear power station at Heysham would be seen
squatting on the horizon straight ahead. Fortunately, my parents' house faced in the opposite direction, towards the Lune
estuary. On a clear day you could spot Blackpool Tower from
their bedroom. I had not lived at home since I had started at
Manchester University. Stepping through the front door was
like stepping back in time. It was impossible to pretend that I
had never been a spotty schoolboy and a stroppy student here.
In those days my mother and father had known me better
than I had known myself. Not any more, though.

The air was cleaner in Lancaster. Its citizens walked at a
slower pace. The pulsating pressure that, depending on your
mood, either energised or enervated you in the capital was
absent here. It was a good place to unwind. I knew that I was
in need of a rest but still missed going to the gym. I had
recently done fifteen minutes on the rowing machine for the
first time. An instructor who had been watching suggested I
might like to train for the national championships: 'You're
one of the best rowers at this gym.' I would have laughed if I
had not been so out of breath. I was flattered and astonished
but had no interest in competing. Exercise already took up too
much of my life.

My father had retired as soon as he was fifty-five but my
mother, who was three years younger, continued to work as

an estate agent. He had hated spending his days with his fingers in other people's mouths. My mother, on the other hand, enjoyed invading people's privacy: it was the only way to value someone's home. Her days were filled with sights of squalor and splendour: damp bedrooms and filthy bathrooms in Morecambe, picture windows and prize-winning gardens in Bolton-le-Sands. In the morning she could be having coffee beside a kidney-shaped swimming pool in Silverdale and dodging owls in Heysham in the afternoon. The birds' owners had converted their knocked-through lounge into a Gothic fantasy: electric flambeaux flickering on the walls, polystyrene gravestones, painted grey, littering the floor. An open window into an aviary at the back allowed the owls to fly in and out at will. There was a cage of white mice in the kitchen.

After dropping off my bag at the house my father and I caught the train to Carnforth. I had a look round the second-hand bookshop and was delighted to find a copy of *A Memorial Service* by J. I. M. Stewart. I already had the other four parts of his Oxford quintet, known overall as *A Staircase in Surrey*. I had been obsessed with Oxbridge ever since I had failed to get in to St John's College, Cambridge, in 1981. Twenty-two of us had sat the entrance examinations: everyone passed except me and another boy. I had always had doubts about my own intellect. I suspected that my third-class body housed a second-class brain. 'And what makes you think you can get in?' asked my father, furious that I had not consulted him about staying on for the extra, seventh, term. It meant that I would not be going to university until the following year. The bad tidings arrived on Christmas Eve. I would be going to

Manchester after all. My father seemed to love me and have a low opinion of me at the same time. 'The boy's a buffoon!' was his constant refrain. No wonder I had lacked self-confidence.

My mother, who had been unable to take the morning off work, joined us at 1pm. We had lunch in a canalside pub. The post office had issued a set of stamps celebrating the bicentenary of the British canal network that morning. The *Stonechat* was not featured. However, I sent Drew a card with all four stamps on the envelope. The card showed an autumnal view of the Ashton Memorial, built by Lord Ashton in memory of his wife. 'England's grandest folly' was all most people saw of Lancaster as they cruised past on the M6. I had played rugby and cricket in its shadow at school and climbed to the top of it several times. Inside the card I simply wrote: 'Miss you madly!'

The following day I sent Drew another card, this time showing John O'Gaunt's Gate, Lancaster Castle. Drew liked castles. His book of British castles was now in the kitchen at Packington Street. The horseshoe set in the centre of the crossroads between Market Street and Penny Street was said to have come from John O'Gaunt's horse. I always stepped on it for luck. I had written the card at midnight, when my father's birthday was finally over. It had been a long day. We had been for a walk through Happy Mount Park in Bare, where childhood holidays had been spent paddling and playing crazy golf with my father's parents – and the illuminations had never been as good as Blackpool's – and been out for dinner with my sister, my grandmother and my godfather,

Frank. The jazz-loving librarian was a genius at finding out-of-print books. He and my father had been friends ever since they had met at school in the 1950s.

'Dear Drew,' I wrote. 'I've been wearing the Calvin Kleins and Timberlands you bought me tonight. They fit perfectly which is great because I've felt close to you all evening. Be grateful you weren't with me: a smoky pub; bad food; cheap wine. Boredom. I can't wait to come home. In fact, when you read this, I'll see you tomorrow. Yippee!' I was fond of my family but found being with them frustrating. I had nothing in common with them except history. We did not, apparently could not, talk about important things. My grandmother's illness was mentioned only once: she would have to wait another month before starting her course of radiotherapy at Christie's in Manchester. I was thankful I had joined BUPA years ago. The word 'cancer' may not have been uttered but it had hung in the air between us. Pretending it did not exist would not make it go away.

When I got back there was no milk in the fridge or bread in the pantry. 'I've been really busy,' explained Drew. 'I've been living off British Rail sandwiches.' It confirmed my suspicions: the boy needed looking after. We fell into the roles of housekeeper and breadwinner. Drew went out to work, I stayed at home and did the shopping, laundry and cleaning. When he left the office Drew would call from Reading or Paddington to tell me he was on his way back. I could then time dinner accordingly. He would come trudging up the stairs – 'Hi, honey, I'm homo!' – I would come out of the kitchen and we would embrace on the landing. It was the best moment of the day.

There were times when I wondered if Drew needed a surrogate mother more than a lover. After all, back in March, he had given me a set of six liqueur glasses on Mother's Day. I later put this down to my insecurity, not his. He had rescued me from Shakespeare Walk and took just as much care of me as I did of him. Lovers were supposed to look after each other, that was what they did. I simply had not experienced it before. We were both strangers to domestic bliss.

The only cloud on the horizon was the question of Drew's residency. Mad Mary had had second thoughts about marrying him. We had tried not to appear too relieved. She would never have coped with sudden visits from the immigration authorities or withstood the inevitable interrogations: 'Whose toothbrush is this?', 'How many nights a week does your husband stay here?', 'Where does he keep his underpants?' The thought of losing Drew to bureaucratic bigotry, or, for that matter, to anything else, filled me with dread.

I continued to review books for the *Independent* and started to research my next novel. The success of my book on *Inspector Morse* had enabled me to acquire an agent, and not just any agent: Carole Blake was one of the best in the business. With her on my side it seemed I could not lose.

Audacious Perversion had been my third novel. The first two, *Channel-Hopping* and *Love Kills*, were gathering dust at the bottom of my wardrobe. Carole told me to add *Audacious Perversion* to the pile. While it would not be difficult to find a publisher for it, the book was not big enough to launch a career. I should try to come up with a novel that was commercial enough to establish me in the marketplace, she wrote. 'You've got real talent and I think it deserves an audience': I blushed when I read the letter. It was wonderful to know that someone had faith in me.

One way to sell a novel was to write an excellent 'treatment', a four-part proposal comprising an introduction, character profiles, synopsis and statement of intent. The document should convince a publisher that the book was not only well worth writing, and therefore buying, but that the writer was capable of delivering it too. Such a commercial approach was new to me. I had naïvely expected to write what I wanted and then let someone else sell the result. That, however, was not how the world worked. You had to earn the right to produce what you wanted: in the meantime you had to write what other people wanted to read. When I had established a devoted following I would be able to dust off *Audacious Perversion* and it would do well. Until then I had to learn the bestselling trade.

Cliffhanger, my first attempt at a high-concept story, had got stuck in San Francisco. The plot worked but the characters were not credible. It needed a lot more work. Meanwhile, Brian, the Film Editor at *Time Out*, told me a true story. His father had been a police constable in the City of London. It was a fascinating tale that immediately gripped my imagination. Brian had known it would. *Snow Hill* would be set in the 1930s. I started researching the period with glee.

My life settled down into a regular routine of gym,

housework and reading. 'It's the life of Riley,' said Geoff when I told him. The *bon viveur* knew little about training or domestic chores. Nevertheless, his tone carried more disapproval than envy. I did not see much of Drew during the week because our days were out of sync: he was already at work when I got up at 8am and had been in bed for a couple of hours when I retired at midnight. However, we spoke on the phone at least once a day and made up for it at the weekend – if he did not have to work. We usually went out on Saturday night or had friends round for dinner. We liked serving drinks on the terrace and using our new Danish dining chairs. The pale beechwood went well with Alex's old table. Sometimes we would finish clearing up after the night before only to immediately start preparing Sunday lunch for Mandy and Henry or Pascal and Marta who were now house-hunting in London. Monday morning hangovers were often the worst.

If, midweek, Drew was able to catch an earlier train, we would meet in the West End to see a film or a play. At the beginning of October, a couple of days after our first 'anniversary' – it was a year since we had met at the Barbican – we went to see *The Baby of Mâcon* at the Lumière cinema in St Martin's Lane. Peter Greenaway, the director, had become a technocrat rather than an auteur. The climactic, epic rape scene was boring rather than horrifying. It was a film in which people mainly moved furniture about. I hailed a cab. I was so busy pontificating that I had not noticed Drew's silence.

'Cat got your tongue?' I put my hand on his leg and rubbed his thigh. He brushed it off. 'What's the matter?'

'Why couldn't we have gone for a drink?'

'I didn't know you wanted to. I thought you'd be ready for bed.' I glanced at the driver. The glass partition was ajar. I slid it shut.

'You never take me to the Groucho any more.'

'Drew, we can go there any time you wish. What's brought this on?'

'I feel cheated. I like to be seen with you. When we go out together we just sit in the dark.'

A week later we were in Heaven. It was *Time Out*'s twenty-fifth birthday party. I had not intended to go but it was the perfect opportunity to show Drew that I was not embarrassed to be seen with him. We bumped into Mandy and Henry in the crowd. I introduced Drew to my old colleagues whenever I could – the difference in our heights must have made us seem an odd couple but I did not care. Drew was delighted to see Michael Palin. He was a big Monty Python fan too. Jeremy Beadle, the television prankster, had found a pocket umbrella outside the cloakroom. He wandered about asking people if it was theirs. 'Does this belong to you?' 'No,' I replied. 'Is it going to explode?' The bearded wonder was not, oddly enough, game for a laugh.

The Diaries of Kenneth Williams had been published that year. I continued to plough my way through them even though, in spite of the odd moment of hilarity, they formed the most depressing book I had ever read. The silly, wise, old queen made me appreciate my own good fortune. One autumnal afternoon I looked up from the page. I was sitting on one of the new sofas that had finally arrived. There was a momentary lull in the rush-hour traffic. The gilt frame of the mirror that hung between the bookshelves glowed in the setting sun. I was waiting for Drew to come home. My God. I was actually happy! That night I wrote in my diary: 'I realised today that this is one of the very best periods of my life – anything can happen.'

On 26 October Drew discovered a swelling on the left side of his groin.

6

GHOSTS

'It's not surprising water's coming in,' said the builder. 'You've got a hole in the roof . . . or might as well have. There's forty broken slates up there at least. Those aerial blokes don't care where they put their feet.' He scratched his head. The stupidity of other people was amazing. 'How're you fixed tomorrow morning?'

'I'll be here.' Apart from the gym, I had nowhere else to go.

The crack across the ceiling of Drew's bedroom was bordered by a pale brown stain. A bucket collected the drips when it rained. If the flat had been empty for three years, and the carpet was not marked, the damage must have been new. The computer was set up in Drew's room but, as I tried day after day to breathe life into the characters in *Cliffhanger*, I had not heard anyone clambering around. I was not having much success with the novel: something was missing. However, the amount of time and effort I had invested in the book made me reluctant to drop it.

Drew had settled in well at Thames Water. A couple of his colleagues had become friends. One of them, Aron, took him to a gym in the City: Drew was so impressed he joined it the following week. 'I was putting on weight, anyway. I didn't realise champagne was so fattening.' He would either attend an aerobics class in the morning or work out in the evening on his way home. I saw even less of him now, an average of just ninety minutes a day.

It was a marriage of sorts. Our social life followed much the same course as the previous year. This new sense of continuity, of permanence, was deeply satisfying. We went to a bonfire party in Wraysbury, hosted by a former Heddonist, and danced round a field waving sparklers as jets from Heathrow took off overhead. Mary was too drunk to drive back so Drew chauffeured us home while she snored on the back seat. It was the first time I had been driven by Drew. He did not have a car and I did not drive. He was confident behind the wheel but I would never have guessed that he was such a speed merchant. We did not notice the camera flash.

We went to see David Hare's *The Absence of War* at the National. John Thaw was magnificent as the embattled Labour leader but there was a total absence of drama. One line, however, did strike home: 'Tragedy is a posh word for losing.' We went to Part II of the American Art in the Twentieth Century exhibition at the Saatchi & Saatchi gallery. I loved the exuberance of Keith Haring; Howard and Sarah laughed at the kitsch of Jeff Koons. Drew bought a postcard of his floating basketball (*One Ball Total Equilibrium Tank*). This was how Sunday afternoons were supposed to be spent: wandering round galleries with other young couples.

Drew insisted we take Howard and Sarah to see *The Winter's Tale* at the Barbican. It was just as enjoyable the second time round. The story of jealousy, forgiveness and a return from the dead had made a deep impression on him.

The four of us celebrated my birthday in style. Amberley Castle in West Sussex declared itself to be 'the friendliest castle in the world'. The 900-year-old ruin had been converted into a luxury hotel. Drew took the Friday off work. He went to the doctor – his lump had yet to disappear – then went on a recce of a dubious polytechnic in Hackney. If he could not marry his way into the country, he would study his way in. Overseas students were also eligible for visas.

After lunch Howard and Sarah picked us up in a Ford Mondeo hired specially for the occasion. We bunny-hopped our way out of South London then hared off down the M23. Drew filmed the sunset from the back seat. 'The Arrival of the Queen of Sheba' was playing on the radio as we approached the raised portcullis and pulled into the spotlit central courtyard. Howard drove round and round on the gravel until the music had finished. 'It's like being back at EuroDisney,' said Drew. My cynicism was beginning to rub off on him.

He, on the other hand, had changed me for the better. If going to Manchester instead of Cambridge had knocked the corners off me, Drew smoothed down the rough edges. He did not judge people by their appearance, he was not quick to condemn. He was more likely to give someone the benefit of the doubt rather than the cold shoulder. His Christian faith, and faith in me, provided us both with an anchor. As I relaxed into the relationship I slowly unfurled. His love gave me confidence, persuaded me, at long last, that I was not irredeemable. He was my life-saver. It was possible to change your life by yourself, but it was easier if you let other people help you.

There is a thin line between confidence and complacence. Still negotiating new territory, I was unaware that I had crossed it. The moment you think you have it all – lover, home, career – is the moment you start to lose it.

We checked in to the hotel and had afternoon tea in front of a crackling, wheezing log fire. Drew said he was feeling tired and went to have a lie down. Our room was at the top of a turret – I had already banged my head on one of the low exposed beams – yet there was still space for a Jacuzzi in the bathroom. We tried it out before dinner while sharing a complimentary bottle of champagne.

'Do you love me?' The question came out of the blue. I could not have been more shocked if he had punched me in the face.

'Of course I do. You know I do.' I put down my glass. 'Why d'you ask?' I held out my hand for his glass but he continued to hold it.

'I think you're grateful. Look at the life you lead. You couldn't do it without me. Gratitude's not the same as love.'

'I know that – and I am grateful – but that doesn't mean I don't love you. I will never forget what you've done for me.

I wouldn't have let you do it if I hadn't felt the same way about you. How can you doubt me? What do I have to do to convince you? Come here.' Drew handed over his glass then slid beside me. I gave him a hug. 'I love you more than I have ever loved anyone. I don't want anybody else. I see other boys at the gym but I don't fancy them any more. It's just window-shopping. The thought of having sex with anyone but you scares the hell out of me.'

It was true. I had finally learned that getting to know one body in great detail, the myriad ways it feels, smells and reacts – and the person inside it – was far more rewarding than any number of torrid flings. It was the difference between making love and making out. Drew was full of surprises. Only that week he had told me that he had once been a marshal at Wembley. He had taken a series of odd jobs soon after arriving in Britain. While it was easy enough to imagine him working behind the counter of a café in Holborn, it was rather more difficult to picture him controlling crowds of rowdy football supporters. Then again, he had taught Australian adolescents. He had many talents. He never bored me. And the knowledge that I had the rest of my life to get to know him properly filled me with joy.

Drew, however, appeared not to know how I felt. I may not have told him, but I had shown him. At least I thought I had. After years of rejection, though, a part of me was still holding back and Drew sensed it. I sometimes thought he knew me better than I did myself. The TVP fiasco had made me determined not to be hurt again. Deep down I was afraid of giving my all to another person. Total surrender was dangerous. I had to convince him that, as things stood, I loved him as much as I could.

'How long have you been thinking about this? You should have said. I've told you before, you can ask me anything.'

'I thought you'd be mad at me.'

'Don't I show you enough affection? Is that it?'

'Nooooo . . . You never say you love me though.'

'I didn't realise I had to. I thought it was obvious.' It was strange how one simple phrase of three little words was so difficult to say when you meant it. However, there was something wrong, something missing, if Drew still had his doubts. We lived together but had separate rooms: it was important to retain some personal space, a degree of independence. Drew wanted us to lose ourselves in each other, but I felt it was still too soon. Our love had not yet been put to the test.

The next morning we were woken by the sound of gravel being thrown at the window. It was the wind dashing raindrops against the diamond-leaded panes. After a full English breakfast we got into the Mondeo and headed for Chichester. Howard, as he drove, hummed along to a Mozart horn concerto. We explored the cathedral, had lunch in a pub then moved on to Bospham where, like King Canute before us, we got our feet wet. Drew bought a model fishing boat; I bought a second-hand copy of *And So to Murder* by Carter Dickson.

The old green Penguin edition felt and smelt so much better than a modern paperback. It was the tag-line on the cover that caught my attention: 'Death in a film studio.' Our flat in Packington Street was only a short walk from the Gainsborough Studios, where Alfred Hitchcock had made his first feature, *The Lodger*, starring Ivor Novello. The locals had dubbed Poole Street 'Hollywood by the Canal'. I was unearthing lots of nuggets of local lore as I researched the background to *Snow Hill*. Dickson's detective story about a vicar's daughter who becomes a scriptwriter for Albion Films might provide some authentic details of movie-making in the 1930s. Besides, the 'half-pint of vitriol poured down a speaking tube' sounded intriguing.

The Roman villa at Bignor, much to Drew's disappointment, was closed. The windscreen-wipers maintained their relentless, deadening rhythm. It was impossible to hear it without being transported back to the endless car-bound afternoons of wet weekends and childhood holidays. Howard, to a chorus of 'Bugger Bignor!', took a detour past Butlin's and on to Ford Open Prison. That night, after a dinner of anchovy mousse, quail salad, poussin with celeriac and walnuts, kirsch sabayon, and several bottles of wine, we braved the pouring rain to peer into the dungeon at midnight.

The walls of Amberley Castle are nine feet thick in parts. As it tore round them, the howling wind sounded almost human. 'It's Emily!' said Drew. A waiter had told us the old, old story of the poor girl who, carrying the local vicar's child, had thrown herself off the top of the gatehouse. Her unquiet spirit was said to haunt the battlements. We staggered to bed.

Our dormer window blew open at 4am. The crash woke both of us up. Cold air blasted into the room. I turned on a bedside lamp. Drew sat bolt upright in his bed and stared out into the darkness. His face was bone-white. 'No!'

'It's all right. It's all right. It's just the wind. Go back to sleep.' I got out of my bed and closed the window, making sure that it could not swing open again. The cold, not fear, raised goosebumps on my skin. It was our last night away together.

'So there you are. Glad you could make it. Come in and liven things up.' Alex was drunk. He had turned thirty the day before. A birthday party was the perfect opportunity to show off his new home in Chiswick. Most of the guests were doused in CK but the aftershave could not quite mask the scent of fresh paint. We followed him down the hall and into the kitchen. Alex pointed at the champagne. A freckle-faced Irish boy tugged at his sleeve. Alex sighed: 'It's about time you bought your own, you know.' They went upstairs.

'Hello.' It was Steven. We had not spoken since Alex's last birthday party. Drew spotted Johnny and went over to chat with him. 'Still together then?'

'Miracles do happen . . . although I was wishing they didn't this afternoon.'

Drew had given me a watch for my birthday. It was big and chunky and had lots of functions. I did not like it. Drew was offended when I asked if he would mind if I changed it for something simpler and slimmer. I had known he would be, but he would have been hurt even more had I never worn the thing. I did my best to be diplomatic. Drew, however, thought I should keep the watch because he had chosen it. He eventually agreed to return to Selfridges and help me choose another one. Besides, we needed to buy some new plates. I was planning a grand dinner party to mark his twenty-ninth birthday. I wanted to show him how much I loved him.

I swapped the fancy, cutting-edge chronometer for a watch that could have been designed in the 1930s. It had a clear, elegant face and weighed much less than its predecessor. I used to wear a watch everyday but stopped in a futile attempt to reduce stress. I was always checking the time. Punctuality was important to me: I was constantly afraid of being late. The strap around my wrist had come to feel like a handcuff. Drew was particularly attracted to men's wrists. My father wore his watch on the inside of his wrist, as if he did not want anyone else to know the correct time, as if he owned the rights to Time itself: 'It's to protect the face, you silly boy.' I was right-handed yet still wore a watch on my right wrist. It seemed natural enough to me. In the end, tired of trying to explain, I said it was so any opponent in a fight would expect me to hit them with my left. I had sat through lots of Saturday morning westerns with my father.

We ambled round and round the basement of the department store. There was a dazzling range of designs on display but Drew was at his most pernickety and we left empty-handed. We trudged through the crowds of Christmas shoppers to Heal's in Tottenham Court Road where Drew found a service that he liked. The blue and gold plates cost £45 each. I refused to pay – could not pay – so much. We needed to buy other items as well – cutlery, for example – as I was determined the dinner party should be the best one I had ever given. The whole afternoon had been a thoroughly dispiriting experience.

'The bad times mean just as much as the good times,' said Steven. 'Believe me.' John, his partner, had died of Aids in August, on the Glorious Twelfth. Alex had told me but I had done nothing. I had never met John. A part of me had wanted to – I wanted to see what he had that I lacked – but most of me did not. However, I was glad that Steven had found someone who made him happy.

'I'm sorry about John. I suppose you're sick of people telling you "'Tis better to have loved and lost than never to have loved at all." Is it true?'

'Most of the time.' He looked away. Steven had made me cry in the past but I had never seen him shed a tear. His eyes remained dry.

'I think you're very brave. I wouldn't be here if I were in your place.'

'It's not bravery when you have no choice. What am I going to do? Stay at home for the rest of my life?'

'Sounds good to me. Why is it so difficult to have fun when you're supposed to be having a good time? Look at them all: pretty boys and ugly queens bickering and boozing, hating themselves as much as each other. Infinite bitches in a little room. "This is hell nor am I out of it."'

'Speak for yourself. I may be a queen but I'm not ugly. I might as well be miserable here as anywhere else.' He drained his glass. 'Drew seems happy enough.'

'He and Johnny have bonded. They both think they're badly treated – and I haven't dumped Drew. Has Johnny met his replacement yet?'

'I think his replacement has already been replaced.'

The next Saturday Drew returned from Reading with wonderful news. His computer agency had agreed to sponsor him. A work visa would allow him to stay in Britain for another three years. He would not have to go through the farce of an arranged marriage nor tire himself out studying for a worthless degree. Our rejoicing was mixed with heart-felt relief. It was proof that we were meant to be together. Drew decided to go home for Christmas: 'I have to tell everyone that my future lies in England.'

I had been looking forward to our first Christmas. However, he deserved a long holiday. A month's separation was nothing compared with three more years together. His birthday dinner would now be even more of a celebration. When I rang Howard to tell him he told me that he and Sarah were going through 'a bad patch' but refused to elaborate. Marriage was out of the question: 'We'll come to your wedding instead.'

There was no sign of tension between Howard and Sarah when they came round to Packington Street for the dinner party. It had taken me a fortnight to prepare for the occasion. The house was spotless: even the windows had been cleaned. It had cost me £25 to have them done inside and out. When I said I was trying to write a thriller the lanky lad had told me he did the 'winduz' for Ken Follett — and Tina Turner and Kylie Minogue too.

There was no space for a Christmas tree so I had bought some twisted willow and decked its boughs with baubles. The black vase and golden balls matched the frame of the living-room mirror perfectly. The black-and-white striped sofas echoed the black-and-white linocuts that hung above them. Mandy had given them to us as a house-warming present. The square one opposite the windows showed Beowulf wrestling with Grendel: 'The waves roughened and the creatures of the deep were lashed into fury/Some fearful monster took hold of me and dragged me to the bottom;/However, I had the luck to get at the brute with the tip of my sword/And in the hurly-burly I dispatched it.' The rectangular pair opposite the bookshelves illustrated extracts from 'The Trees' by Philip Larkin. Everything was as it should be. The stage was set.

After a couple of bottles of Bollinger we all transferred to the kitchen. Geoff sat at the head of the table. Howard and Sarah faced Drew and I. Cooking in front of people always made me nervous but the champagne helped. There were, miraculously, no disasters. I served Muscadet with the tomato and orange soup; a white Hermitage with the scallops, salmon and monkfish in herb butter; a 1985 Hermitage with the roast partridge with juniper; and a Chénas with the cheese. The dessert came in a large white box. I asked Drew to take off the lid.

His birthday cake had been baked in the shape of Australia and covered in terracotta icing. Cairns was marked in big black letters; Sydney, Canberra, Perth and Darwin in smaller ones. It reminded me of the map Drew had drawn in his reply to my Lonely Hearts ad. Uluru dominated the Red Centre near Alice Springs; Hobart lay off the southern coast in a blue and silver Tasman Sea; Sydney was represented by its opera house. A kangaroo pointed to a plaque in the left-hand corner: 'Good Luck Drew'. He gave me a hug.

Howard took photos as Drew cut the cake. We wished him Bon Voyage, Happy Birthday and Merry Christmas. We washed the sponge down with a glass of dessert wine then returned to the living room where there was coffee, chocolates, port and marrons glacés for those who wanted them. It was almost 3am when, clutching presents, our guests finally staggered to their taxis. I cleared away most of the debris. The washing up, however, would have to wait till the morning.

Drew came out of the bathroom as I dragged myself up the stairs. We kissed on the landing. 'Thank you, Sweetie. You surpassed yourself.'

'Glad you enjoyed it. I do love you, Drew.'

'I know.'

I wrote my Christmas cards while Drew did his packing. I gave him two parcels to take with him: one contained an Armani belt for his birthday, the other was his Christmas box. It comprised a miniature kaleidoscope, a pair of cufflinks that read HOT and COLD, an atomiser, a silver credit-card case, a pen that wrote upside down, a bar of chocolate, a keyring, a pack of cards and a matt brass photo-frame with a picture of me (taken at Amberley Castle) inside. They were all individually wrapped so, in addition, I gave him a list of the contents in a sealed envelope to hand to any overzealous customs officer. I also slipped a card into his suitcase: 'Missing me yet?'

On the Sunday morning we took a cab to King's Cross then got the Tube to Heathrow. Fairy lights blinked in every direction. Richard Branson worked his way along the line, glad-handing passengers and apologising for the queue. Our brief farewell was downbeat. I watched Drew walk through the departure gate. He did not look back.

The flat seemed empty without him. It was too big for one person. I wandered from room to room, up and down the stairs, catching things out of the corner of my eye. On the first night I lay in his bed, breathing his scent off the pillow, but went to my own room before falling asleep. When I got up on Tuesday morning there was a message from Drew on the answerphone. It had taken him forty-one hours to get home. He called again at 11pm when it was already his birthday. It was good to hear his voice.

I was not alone for long: my parents came to visit. They were impressed by the flat. 'How can you possibly afford to live here?' asked my father. 'Drew earns a lot more than me,' I replied. They slept in Drew's room. I took my mother to see *Crazy for You* at the theatre but they had to amuse themselves for the rest of their stay because I was busy previewing programmes for the *Sunday Times* again.

On their last night in London I took my parents to the Groucho Club to have dinner with Howard and Sarah and Alison, a friend who worked in radio. 'You can be my beard,' I told her. 'I'm sure Drew wouldn't mind you taking his place.' I did, though. I was being forced to play a role again, pretending I was someone I was not. I missed Drew even more than I had expected: I felt his absence like an amputee feels his missing limb. It physically hurt. And denying his importance in my life only made the pain worse. The thought of my mother and father sitting round a table with Drew and I, eating and drinking and laughing, accepted and accepting, was seductive, but I doubted that it could ever be achieved. Denholm Elliott, the actor, had died earlier that year. 'You'd never have known he was queer,' said my mother. She did not realise the insulting adjective had been reclaimed by gay militants.

After that, Christmas followed the usual routine. I gave Howard his annual lesson in how to do *The Times* crossword on the train to Lancaster; my grandmother came to stay on Christmas Eve. I was still wrapping presents in front of *Chitty Chitty Bang Bang* when she arrived with enough luggage for a month. I had collected her present to me from Waterstone's that morning: the new edition of the *Shorter Oxford English Dictionary*. I had already opened Drew's present. The fluffy, white bathrobe from Liberty had been too big to transport. The card inside quoted R. Maria Rilke on the front: 'For one human being to love another . . . that is perhaps the most difficult of all our tasks, the final and ultimate proof, the task for which all others are but preparation.' So I was not the only one who found it difficult to love and be loved.

Drew called at 12.15pm on Christmas Day. He must have heard the first champagne cork pop. It was 10.15pm in Cairns. He had a sinus infection, and sunburn, but his mother was looking after him. The flight from Brisbane had been uneventful. David, his brother, lived in the Queensland capital. All I knew about him was that he also worked in computers, had a girlfriend called Jan, and used to have standing-on-one-leg competitions with Drew. A postcard had arrived from Brisbane before I left London: 'Sweetie: Miss You, Love You, Together Forever '94!'

We did not watch Quentin Crisp deliver his alternative Queen's Message from New York – even though it had been my idea and Panoptic had produced it. I wanted to hear The Beatles' 'Red Album', which my sister had bought me, but our parents did not have a CD player. Instead, to escape the cigar smoke, the two of us went for a walk. There was a hard frost, a gibbous moon and no one else about. A silent night. Other families, in paper hats, lay bloated on sofas in front of the flickering box. It would have been a good moment to tell Linda about Drew. However, I did not. We talked mainly about our grandmother. The radiotherapy seemed to be working.

I spent New Year's Eve alone, consoling myself that at least Drew was on his way home. After a stopover in Hawaii, he had arrived in Los Angeles where I had arranged for him to have dinner with Laurie, an old friend of mine whom he had met once before. I opened a bottle of champagne, watched Clive James on BBC1, and waited for my parents to call at midnight. The year had ended much better than it had started. I put in my ear-plugs and went to bed. The exploding rockets sounded like distant gunfire.

A land mine had destroyed the terrace behind Packington Street during the Second World War. It came down on a parachute but went off before it hit the ground. If you looked at the front of some of the houses in the street, you could see where the walls still bulged because of the blast. Kids played on the bombsite for years. Then they built the council flats.

The Fenerons had lived in Packington Street for forty years. Most of them had been spent at Number 29 but they had been happy to shift a few doors down when they saw how nicely they had done the place out. 'We looked at your flat,' said Elsie. 'Too many stairs.' Sometimes, tired of staring at the computer, or fed up with being alone, I would pop down for a chat. I liked hearing about Islington's unglamorous past. Arthur had retired from Faraday's near Highbury Corner but he kept himself busy pottering about. He sometimes sat on the front steps in the sun, smoking a roll-up and watching the world go by. He had been captured in Singapore and sent to work on the Burma Railway. He showed me the scars where the bamboo slashes had ulcerated. 'I've never dreamed about it. Not once.'

I was embarrassed when Elsie said, soon after we moved in, 'If you need any shopping doing just let me know. It's difficult when you've both got jobs.' I thanked her but did not take her up on the offer. She was a senior citizen. We should have been shopping for her. I was even more embarrassed one morning when, casting a quizzical glance up at the house, she said: 'You don't do your windows do you?' I spent the afternoon calling window-cleaners. I blushed to think what they said about the garden. It was all right for them: their half had been paved.

The couple were happy to talk about the past. 'We moved in on our wedding day in 1947,' said Elsie. 'Two rooms and a gas-ring on the landing. No bathroom. The Hicks had your place. She died of cancer, poor thing. Only young she was.' The fact that Drew and I lived together did not seem to bother them. One of their daughters had emigrated to Australia. Rosemary lived in Hastings, near Melbourne. They went out to see her and the grandchildren whenever they could.

Drew arrived home at dusk on 2 January. I brought one of his cases into the hall and waited while he paid the driver. He smiled as he came up the steps. He looked browner and happier. I threw my arms around him as soon as the door was closed. We stood there for at least a minute. 'Let me get my coat off then.' I did not want to let go.

I tried on my new T-shirts as the bathtub filled. There was a present from Hawaii too, a set of six raku coasters decorated with petroglyphs: Man on Surfboard, Running Man, Spear Man. As I climbed into the water Drew said 'that's the best sight I've seen in weeks'. There were no bubbles left when we got out. We shared a bottle of champagne and watched the first part of Barbara Vine's *A Dark-Adapted Eye* on television. Drew fell asleep on my shoulder.

He slept till after 5pm the next day. The gym had re-opened after the Christmas break but I stayed at home, unwilling to leave him. It was so quiet I met a mouse in the kitchen. It was hard to say who was more surprised. I often watched the sooty mice darting about the suicide pit beneath the live rail on the Underground. This, however, was too close for comfort. I did not scream but I did leap on to a chair. It could have been up my trouser leg in seconds. I found a hole down the side of the washing machine, and got Drew to block it up.

His postcard from Waikiki, posted in Honolulu on New Year's Eve, arrived a few days later. 'The people are very friendly,' concluded Drew, 'but I'll tell you about that in person.' I was sure Drew would have had plenty of opportunities to be unfaithful. He had mentioned a Californian psychologist called Nathan several times. They had, apparently, hung out together in Hawaii. If the photographs were anything to go by, his main talent was for putting a finger in front of the lens. 'He's got a boyfriend,' said Drew. 'So have you,' I replied. I knew Drew loved me but it was hard to believe that he still found me attractive. If he felt the need to play away sometimes, so be it — as long as he continued to come home. I could not decide if such an attitude was adult or stupid.

The telephone stopped ringing. It was as if I had been forgotten. The first month was a time to knuckle down, to work off debts, but I was finding it very difficult to get work. *Cliffhanger* joined *Audacious Perversion* at the bottom of the wardrobe. Novels about Aids, no matter how indirectly, were just not sexy. Carole, my agent, liked the sound of *Snow Hill*, however, so I continued researching the period. A season of programmes about the 1930s was broadcast on Radio 3, and I listened to them avidly.

The fourteenth of February fell on a Monday. However, the preceding weekend, members of Drew's gym could bring a free guest with them to celebrate St Valentine's Day. Drew took me.

It was a different world. The vast gym, thirty times bigger than N16, was underneath the arches of Cannon Street Station, next door to LIFFE, the London International Financial Futures Exchange. It was where the Big Swinging Dicks of the City hung out – but not on a Sunday afternoon. The large, luxurious changing rooms were virtually deserted. The lockers and carpet put the hooks and lino of N16 to shame. There was a 25m swimming pool as well. Then again, it cost twice as much to join.

The free weights room and work-out studios were much busier. Drew joined me in the sauna after his aerobics class. I was far more relaxed than I had been in Nice – although the strange surroundings, and sheer size of the place, were daunting at first. It was good to see some new faces, and bodies, as well.

'Thanks for bringing me. I'd have been worried about

bringing my boyfriend to such a macho gym.' Drew laughed. He looked round the café.

'It's not as if we're the only ones.'

It snowed on the day itself. A large card arrived from Drew with the stamps stuck on in the shape of a heart. I had left his on the kitchen table the night before. The Keith Haring design showed two dancers holding hands with a heart where their heads should have been. Our circle of friends remained silent. Everyone seemed to have shrunk into themselves. Alex was supposed to bring round his new boyfriend, James Bond – 'No, really, his name is James Bond' – but on the afternoon in question there was no sign of them and no word.

A few days later Drew was ill with an upset stomach. He stayed off work and spent the day in bed. I thought it was indigestion.

'I saw a ghost this morning.' I looked up from my book. I was lying on the sofa-bed in his room to keep him company.

'Oh yeah?'

'I knew you wouldn't believe me. There's a cold patch to the right of the door, near to the bookcase. I feel it every morning when I get up. It was in exactly the same place. I wasn't dreaming.'

'What did it look like?'

'Hazy, shimmering, blue. I wasn't scared.'

'Male or female?'

'Male.' Good. I had not told him about the Hicks.

'And?'

'Well, he was shortish, dark, young I think. He went through the wall into the bathroom. It was only when he started to turn his head that I got the willies. I thought he was going to look right at me but he faded away before I could see his face.'

'Fetch' is an old English word for a ghost. The *Concise Oxford Dictionary* defines it as 'the apparition or a double of a living person, believed to be a warning of that person's impending death'. In other words, the fetch, if that is what Drew saw, had come to get him. At the time I did not believe in such things. I do now.

7

FRENCH FARCE

Drew's vision soon took on the status of a portent as our luck began to run out. Nothing went right. It was as if the man in the control-room had decided that he was not directing a romantic drama but a French farce. We, like Jason and the athletic granny, would have to negotiate a long and difficult assault course.

Perhaps Drew, when he got up on 1 March, did not say 'white rabbits'. His inquiries about a job at the Angel led to a threat from his agency to rescind the application for a three-year visa. The computer industry, like any other, thrived on inside information. Changing agencies was tantamount to treason. It would have been great for Drew to walk to work in ten minutes rather than travel to Reading every day – the journey never took less than an hour, even if he caught a cab to Paddington – but he withdrew from the running immediately. The next day he was told that his mollified agency had applied for a four-year working visa instead.

However, there was a catch. It would take between four and six weeks to complete the necessary paperwork which meant that, because his current visa expired on 28 March, Drew would have to be put on a temporary visa in the meantime. He was required to surrender his passport to the Home Office. We were due to fly to Brussels on the 29th because the law required you to be out of the country on the day a new visa came into effect. The trip was intended to be a spring break, a temporary reprieve from the daily grind courtesy of Air Miles. If we cancelled because Drew did not have his passport, we would lose the hard-earned loyalty rewards. Howard, who would be on his Easter holiday by then, agreed to come with me instead.

Drew also had to be able to prove that he was out of the country on the day that the application for his new visa was made, so on 10 March we took the 8.33 stopping train to Dover. It was a relief when the castle finally came into view. The train stopped at the station beneath it. 'Change here for the ferry terminal,' called a guard who was sauntering along the platform. 'The courtesy bus will be here in a minute.' It never turned up. We, and another furious couple, eventually shared a cab to the terminal where those who had stayed on the train had caught the 11.30 ferry to Calais. We had missed it and had to wait for the 12.30 crossing.

Lunch was vile. I had been eighteen the last time I travelled on a cross-channel ferry. Howard and I were returning from Paris on the eve of Prince Charles's wedding to Lady Diana

Spencer. We had trailed round the Louvre, been up and down the escalators of the Pompidou Centre and stared at the rent-boys in the Tuileries. Monet's water lilies, Colbert's canal and Napoleon's tomb had all been ticked off the list. Our hotel had been little better than a flea-pit. The highlight for me was reading *Anna Karenina* in the Luxembourg Gardens, slurping milkshakes from McDonald's in the sun. I had lost my appetite for junk food now.

The ro-ro docked at 2pm GMT. We were the only people on board the bus to the arrivals hall who were not wearing shell-suits. Instead of heading for the hypermarkets, we went back through immigration where Drew's passport received the all-important stamp, got back on the bus and caught the same ferry back to Dover. The duty-free shop was a zoo: trolleys bearing leaning towers of lager collided with pensioners dragging wheelie-baskets stuffed with Ferrero Rocher chocolates, cheap sherry and Bailey's Irish Cream. Outside, thankfully, the sun was shining. I took a photo of Drew against the white cliffs of Dover but this was not a cruise to remember. Crossing the Styx would have been more fun.

We boarded another bus. At Passport Control Drew was given the third degree because his current visa had less than three weeks to run. I could do nothing but stand and wait on the other side of the line, cursing a country that did not legally recognise love between men. If one of us had been female this bureaucratic rigmarole would have been irrelevant. Drew paid British taxes – more than most British citizens – but the British government paid him no respect.

Yet another bus took us back to the station. There was no

heating on the slow train to Victoria and the windows would not stay closed. We could not even find two seats together so we sat and shivered while raucous schoolgirls flung four-letter words at each other. And Drew had chosen to live in this country to be with me.

We went through the front door of Packington Street at nearly half-past seven, twelve hours to the minute since we had left; all for ten minutes on French soil. The telephone was ringing. The cancer had spread to my grandmother's lungs.

The next day Drew told me that he needed an operation. He had been to see his doctor on the way to work, and the diagnosis for the lump in his groin had changed: it was not hardened faeces, as had originally been thought, but a swollen gland. It ought to be removed.

'Why didn't you tell me you'd made an appointment?'

'I didn't want to worry you. It's probably nothing.'

However, the lump began to hurt. Drew was advised to go to the Casualty department at University College Hospital. The doctor who examined him said that he should be operated on within a fortnight. The following day, Friday 18 March, Drew was told he should present himself at UCH on Tuesday. The swiftness of the response did not make us suspicious.

We were not the only ones facing an uncertain future. Pascal was fired from his new job in Paris and Panoptic were in shock. Jean's husband had died in hospital after a routine operation. My grandmother started a course of chemotherapy.

We carried on as if we had all the time in the world. We

booked a converted water-mill near Cognac for the first two weeks in September. I applied for the job of Assistant Film Buyer at Channel 4. In the meantime I continued to research *Snow Hill*. I wanted to prove myself as a writer to Drew.

Jonathan Swift had already provided me with an epigraph to the novel. His poem, 'A City Shower', contains the following lines:

Now from all parts the swelling kennels flow,
And bear their trophies with them as they go:
Filths of all hues and odours, seem to tell
What streets they sailed from, by the sight and smell.
They, as each torrent drives with rapid force
From Smithfield, or St Pulchre's shape their course;
And in huge confluent join at Snow Hill ridge,
Fall from the conduit prone to Holborn Bridge.
Sweepings from butchers' stalls, dung, guts and blood
Dead cats and turnip-tops come tumbling down the
flood

The helter-skelter pace and graphic imagery created exactly the right atmosphere for a local story about dirty deeds in dark places. However, I was so preoccupied with turning reality into fiction that I was blind to what was happening in front of me. I had no idea how messy life could get.

Drew spent most of 22 March waiting to be admitted to hospital, but at 4pm he was sent home with some painkillers.

'They said it would be next week now.' He was angry yet relieved. He did not like needles. I tried to reassure him by saying, 'They wouldn't have postponed the operation if they thought it was serious,' but we both knew that was not true.

The next morning his new working visa arrived. It was for two years, not four – the application for a temporary visa had been a complete waste of time. The second post returned his passport. He could have come to Brussels after all. 'It would be unfair to ask Howard to back out now,' said Drew. 'Besides, the hospital might call while I was away.'

Drew still needed to leave the United Kingdom though. So, on 29 March, he took an early morning flight to Paris whereas Howard and I caught an afternoon flight to Brussels. It was an important day because our future was guaranteed for two more years, but we should have been celebrating together rather than flying out to different countries. Drew sent me a black-and-white postcard of the Passerelle des Arts. There were two people on the footbridge about to pass in the middle. 'Dear Mark, how is Brussels? As I write this I know you are probably already on your way to the airport to catch your plane. Soon I will be doing likewise – but it's back to London for me. It's been a grand day. The only thing to mar my visit is that you weren't here to share it with me. See you soon. Take care. Lots of love, Drew.' It was the last card he ever sent me.

Brussels was a building site. Cranes conducted a stately dance as they feathered new nests for Eurocrats. We worked our way through the galleries of modern and ancient art – hello Dalí, goodbye Rubens; lunched outside in the Grand Place; and wondered why the Mannekin Pis had ever become famous. When I moved into Shakespeare Walk I found a heavy brass corkscrew, a souvenir of Brussels, under one of the kitchen cupboards. Opening a bottle of wine with a little boy's cock was not my idea of a joke. We strolled through the Hubert Arcades and even visited the Tintin museum. I bought Drew a souvenir pair of socks.

There was one thing that I had been determined to do in Belgium. Ever since I had studied W. H. Auden's 'Musée des Beaux Arts' at school I had wanted to see *The Fall of Icarus* with my own eyes. The poem begins: 'About suffering they were never wrong,/The Old Masters'. It ends with the poet contemplating Pieter Bruegel's painting. My heart began to thump as I entered the room. There it was: the 400-year-old masterpiece simply hanging on the wall. As I approached the picture the air seemed to hold its breath, the atmosphere to thicken. The ploughman's shirt was startlingly red. It was easy to miss the drowning: that was the point Bruegel and Auden were making. The ploughman and the shepherd have their backs to Icarus. They do not see his 'white legs disappearing into the green/Water'. His demise means nothing to them:

> and the expensive delicate ship that must have seen
> Something amazing, a boy falling out of the sky,
> Had somewhere to get to and sailed calmly on.

The story of the boy who flew too close to the sun haunted

me. Ambition and guilt were always mixed in my mind. The small voice never stopped asking: 'What makes you think you can do that?' If you did not stick your head above the parapet it would not get shot off. 'Overweening' was such an ugly word. You could not expect other people to care whether or not you achieved your heart's desire. They had their own lives to lead. Icarus failed, so what? His death was just a drop in the ocean.

Drew had still not heard from UCH on Maundy Thursday. He increased his daily dose of Meptazinol to 200mg but it did little to control the pain. I hated not being able to help him. I gave him the Easter egg that I had bought in Brussels.

Drew went to work the next day but came home in the afternoon feeling much worse. I called the doctor's surgery. It was a bank holiday: a locum service was in operation. I almost laughed when I opened the door. A sweet little old lady in a beautiful gold sari stood on the step. It took her such a long time to climb the three flights of stairs to Drew's bedroom I feared she was in need of medical attention herself. He explained his condition and stressed the pain. She prescribed antibiotics. It was, apparently, the best she could do. The drug would fight the infection. I bit my tongue. Drew seemed satisfied enough. The nearest chemist that was open on Good Friday was at Marble Arch. I knew it was a waste of time but went and fetched the pills anyway. The first of April was a day for fools' errands.

We were due to go out for dinner that evening. Drew

refused to cancel. He had recently got back in touch with an old flame – someone he had met through a previous ad in *Time Out*. Drew had not told me much about the time he had spent in England before we met, but I knew that Chris, my predecessor, was a doctor. He worked in a hospice not far from his home in North London. He was tall, dark and handsome. If Drew had a type then we both more or less conformed to it. 'There's nothing to tell,' Drew had said as the cab crawled up Holloway Road. 'It didn't work out, that's all.' He was wearing his HOT and COLD cufflinks and his new Tintin socks. The two other guests were also a couple: Peter, a surveyor, and Derek, an actor. The latter became quite enamoured with Drew. Drew was more interested in the fact that a member of Bananarama lived next door.

We each woke up with a hangover. We went for a walk to clear our heads but Drew had to come home when we reached Islington Green: the pain in his groin was too great. He lay on his bed or on one of the sofas, reading or watching TV. At one stage he was in tears. I did my best to distract him. He was, understandably enough, tetchy at times but he made a much better patient than I would have done. I assured him it was safe to double the dose of the Meptazinol. The crisis had come at the worst possible moment. All we could do was wait.

Sunday was spent in much the same way. We set up the Amiga so Drew could play computer games in bed. As usual I did the Azed crossword in the *Observer*. Cruciverbalism was my secret vice. On a good day it took me less than ten minutes to complete the cryptic one in *The Times*. I even belonged to the Crossword Club, members of which received a monthly newsletter containing two puzzles: one relatively easy and one very hard. The esoteric vocabulary and the wit of the compilers were part of the attraction, but what appealed most about crosswords was the fact that, as long as you put in enough time, they presented problems that could always be solved. Everything in their black-and-white world meant something. Order could be achieved out of chaos.

The Azed crossword also featured a clue-writing competition on the first Sunday of each month. Solvers had to complete the puzzle to discover the word that had to be clued. This month's clue-word was 'death'.

Drew was up for much of the night; he could not sleep for the pain. We lay on his bed holding hands. When Monday evening finally arrived he was nearing the end of his tether.

The local surgery opened at 8.30am. I called at 8.31. The line was, of course, engaged. When I did get through I was informed that Drew's doctor was on holiday. The best course of action was to take Drew back to Casualty at UCH. We got a black cab and were there by 9.15.

I had an interview at Channel 4 an hour later. I promised Drew I would return as quickly as possible. Fortunately the television company was then based nearby in Charlotte Street. I had been surprised to get an interview, but if I ever had any chance of landing the job of Assistant Film Buyer I blew it straight away by blathering on about how I had just taken a friend to hospital round the corner. The interviewers made sympathetic noises. They had a position to fill: Drew's predicament was irrelevant. It would have been a dream existence, travelling the world, watching films and deciding which ones should be shown on Channel 4, but I had no experience of handling rights or budgets. It was unrealistic to expect my first job application to be successful, even if I did know a lot about cinema. Financial problems were not solved that easily.

Drew was sitting in the reception area when I returned. The battered plastic seating, the lift doors pinging open, the ebb and flow of people from all directions: it was like being in a third-world airport. The disappointment was written all over his face. He clutched a white paper bag containing some more pills and a green appointment card. It was six days before the consultant could see him. To make matters worse, it had been assumed, because he was gay, that he was HIV-positive. Doctors were not demi-gods, they were human. They could be bigots too.

The pills did the trick, and Drew returned to work. I went to the gym on alternate mornings and resumed my research on *Snow Hill*. I was almost ready to start writing the treatment.

At about the same time my grandmother had finished her first course of chemotherapy. Our conversations were punctuated with bouts of terrible coughing. Once she started it was difficult to stop. She was bringing up blood now. 'This is your telephone bill, Mark David. I'll get my breath back in a minute.' 'Nana, it doesn't matter. Take your time. Don't try to talk. I'll keep chattering on.' It became increasingly difficult to do so: my mind would go blank. Here was someone else I could not help.

On Sunday evening Drew and I went for dinner in Aden Grove. Mandy was looking after a house which had a large garden at the rear. A hedgehog snuffled about under the apple trees. Henry lit a log fire in the living room. After the meal we settled down around it. Drew lay on a sofa and I sat on the floor beside him. The atmosphere of fond relaxation vanished when Drew put his hand on my shoulder and said, 'I've found another lump.' It was at the base of his neck on the left. He saw the fear in my eyes.

Drew saw Dr Scurr, a UCH vascular surgeon, at 11.15 the following morning. He was to be admitted to the Middlesex Hospital that afternoon. We nosed our way through the maze of corridors like a pair of laboratory mice. Mechanical polishers whirred on every floor. Drew had to have a blood test and a chest X-ray before he could be admitted. We were home by 12.30pm. Two hours later we returned to the Middlesex. There were no beds available. At 5pm Drew was told to come back at 7am the next day. His operation was booked for 8.30.

The alarm went off at 5.30am. We saw the sun rise, the first jumbo rumble over, the streetlights blink off. The dawn chorus petered out as we walked slowly up Packington Street. We were in the Thomson Walker Ward by 6.45. It was two and a half hours before Drew got into a bed. The anaesthetist chatted to him as various forms and disclaimers were completed. Finally, at 9.45, Drew was wheeled up to the theatre. I squeezed his hand goodbye.

I was glad to get out of the hospital. The weeks, days and hours of waiting were over at last. It was not easy doing nothing. Even the pollution in Goodge Street smelled better than the warm, synthetic air of the ward. I felt jet-lagged from the early start, and sick when I thought of strangers slicing into Drew's groin. I caught the Number 73 outside the tube station and shopped in M&S at the Angel before returning home for breakfast. I rang my mother to wish her a happy birthday. At noon I dragged myself to the gym.

The telephone rang at ten to four. 'Hi. It's me.'

'How did it go?'

'I feel okay but the doctor said that it was not an easy op. They've removed the lymph gland. I had some kind of reaction to the anaesthetic and woke up screaming in agony although I don't remember anything about it. They had to give me a morphine enema and two injections in my leg.'

'God. You're such a drama queen.'

I set off through the wind and rain to catch a bus back to the Middlesex. It was odd, unreal somehow, seeing Drew tucked up in a hospital bed. I was relieved when he got dressed. At home I made us something to eat and was glad to see that Drew had not lost his appetite, but he was understandably sleepy and sore so we had an early night.

The results of the biopsy would not be available until Monday. We had five days to wait. Each one seemed to bring more bad news: the tenants of Shakespeare Walk gave notice; I was not called for a second interview at Channel 4; my reviewing work dried up. Drew accompanied me on shopping trips to the Angel, but otherwise rested as much as he could. I did not want to bother him about our money troubles. A five-minute telephone call secured me a £5,000 loan.

The weekend seemed to last for ever. At last, amid the uncertain glory of an April day, we returned to UCH. I spotted two magpies from the back of the cab: 'There you are. One for sorrow, two for joy. I told you it would be good news.' His name was called promptly at 10.15. He disappeared down a corridor; I remained in the fourth-floor waiting room and did the *Times* crossword. It was always easy on a Monday. The plastic fittings and pastel colours already seemed familiar. We had sat in six such places during the past month: different departments, different hospitals, all with the same smell of boredom.

Drew reappeared on the stroke of eleven. He was shaking with fury. I had never seen him so angry. I followed him down the corridor into another waiting area off which led a dozen red doors. It was empty. We sat down on a couple of red chairs. Drew was white. 'I'm going to die. It was malignant. I've got cancer.'

'Don't be ridiculous.' Before I could say anything else Drew was called back into one of the consulting rooms. I was desperate to go to the lavatory. The only one I could see was for disabled patients. I used it anyway. It was not the shock: I had been drinking endless cups of water to counteract a hangover. Tragedy can strike at the most tawdry of moments.

We drank chemical coffee while Dr Cheatle telephoned Dr Duchesne, the consultant oncologist, at the Middlesex. Drew needed two operations and would have to undergo chemotherapy. He was given an appointment on Wednesday. I felt as if I were falling. My heart was plunging down a lift shaft. We walked to Euston and caught a bus to the Angel. We shopped in M&S. Such mundane behaviour seemed preposterous in the circumstances but we had no choice other than to carry on.

Drew called his parents as soon as we got home. 'I'm all right. We'll talk later.' I nearly broke down. The French film *Betty Blue* had recently made me cry – why did I feel the need to fight back tears when the situation justified them in real life? I had to be strong for both of us. Drew would not be able to go to work for months. After lunch I forced myself to sit down and start plotting the outline of *Snow Hill*. Three hours produced twenty-four chapters in two sections of twelve. I realised that removing the first letter of each word in the title spelled out NOW ILL.

We did talk that evening but not about important things. We both needed time to come to terms with the idea of cancer, yet time was the one thing we did not have. I wished it were the other way round. Drew had a low pain threshold. If he was embarrassed to be ill, I felt guilty for being healthy. I could not stop having selfish thoughts: what would happen if he died? All I had ever wanted to do was look after Drew, to see that he came to no harm. I had failed. There was nothing I could do now except carry him through the treatment. He was young, fit, and finally in good hands. He had a lot to live for. The ordeal would bring us closer together, if that were possible. Just when things seemed to be falling into place they had started to fall apart.

He was still awake when I came up to bed. I gave him a Temazepam and cuddled him till he fell asleep. When I got up at eight o'clock he had gone to work. I called him.

'Calm down. I'm all right. There's no point me mooching around at home. I know you find it difficult to write when I'm there.'

It made no difference. I could not think about anything else. I went to the gym then spent the afternoon in a trance. If they had removed the lymph gland why was the lump still there? When Geoff rang I told him the news. Mandy rang soon afterwards: Geoff had called her (they had remained friends even though they were no longer a couple). They were acting out of genuine concern but I did not want to talk about it. It was our business, not theirs.

That evening Drew seemed to have regained his self-possession. The day had gone better than expected. He had only taken a couple of Nurofen after lunch even though he had spent most of the time sitting at his desk. I was not sure I believed him. Meanwhile his colleagues had organised 'The Drew Morgan Operation Sweepstake':

One of our dearest whingeing Aussie contractors, Drew 'Mercenary' Morgan, is currently laid up in a London hospital having a mystery operation. Apparently he had difficulty walking last week, is 'having it out' this week and may return to work by Friday. The challenge is to correctly guess the nature of the operation he is so coy about and Aron will give you his Grand National winnings.

The options ranged from 'superiority complex removal' and 'kangaroo pouch sewn up' to 'didgeridoo cleansing' and 'Dame Edna specs fitting'. Some wag had added 'change of agency'. His friend Aron himself had opted for 'analysis for Olivia Newton-John fixation'.

'And what about your day? Did you get much done?'

'Not really.' Cancer had been in our lives for less than thirty-six hours and yet it appeared we had already lost the ability to communicate. It came down to one thing: we were scared.

The waiting room in the oncology department was orange. It was also full. Patients and their fidgeting partners flicked through magazines, stared at their feet or stole glances at their neighbours. Drew's appointment with the consultant was for 9.30am. We were fifteen minutes early. After all, patients were instructed: 'Please attend at the time stated on your card.' At eleven o'clock Jessica, the staff nurse, told us that his medical notes could not be found. They were eventually traced to UCH. I walked over to fetch them. It was midday when Drew was called in to see a different doctor. The waiting faces slowly changed but the murmuring, sighing and yawning remained constant. I had another cup of coffee and ate a Kit-Kat. It was almost an hour before Drew re-emerged.

It would be a miracle if he were still alive in two years. He told me this in the corridor on the way to the scanner department. I stopped falling and hit rock bottom. He had melanoma: skin cancer. So much for 'Slip, Slop, Slap'. His family had always followed the safe sunbathing code promoted by the Australian government: 'Slip on a T-shirt, slop on some sun-screen and slap on a hat.' He was given an appointment on Friday: two more days to wait. We traipsed round the corner to the blood-test labs in Cleveland Street so that Drew's T-cells could be checked again – he really did hate needles – then walked round to *Time Out*'s new offices in Tottenham Court Road. I did not know what else to do.

Geoff was, mercifully, still there even though it was 1.20pm. So was Brian, who asked me how I was getting on with *Snow Hill*, and Elaine, sporting a trophy tan acquired on a recent African safari. Small talk over, Geoff took us to a brasserie in Charlotte Street. I only cried when Drew went to the lavatory.

The real crying started when we got home. We had, as usual, got the bus to the Angel and shopped at M&S. Drew may have been dying but he still needed to eat. It felt like the end for both of us. He went straight to his room. I followed him up. We held each other as we wept. I had never known such grief. The unfairness, suddenness, sheer bloody-mindedness of it was overwhelming. Why Drew? Why now? Why us? I could feel my heart breaking. 'I don't want to die,' wailed Drew. 'I don't want to die.'

*

Drew rang his parents to tell them the news. He asked me to stay in the room. I waited till he had gone to bed before I called my mother. My grandmother had been coughing so much she had pulled a muscle in her groin. I told her that I was about to find out what they had been going through because Drew had cancer too. She offered me the consolation that he would return to Australia before the very worst came. When I said that I would go with him there was silence.

Drew went to work again the next day. A scrawled note awaited me on the kitchen table:

> Sweetie, I rang Mom and Pop again to check how they were. They seem to be taking it well. More importantly, they have decided not to be rash and so will not be coming over yet. How are you this morning? I feel quite cheesed off but otherwise OK. Ring me if you need to talk. Take care. Love you. Drew.

I remained in a trance. Nothing seemed to matter any more; everything seemed to matter all the more. The sun shone. Jets tore white gashes in the blue silk of the sky.

The evening was the most difficult time. Drew's mood changed by the minute: he was calm, maudlin, giggly, angry, depressed, affectionate and desperate. He was already a different person. I did not want him to become bitter like me. He had been my salvation, now I had to be his. It was impossible for me to love him any more than I did. Whether he lived another twenty years or just twenty months, our past could not be taken away from us. In the meantime, no matter what happened, we had each other. The rest of the world could go hang.

Friday arrived at last. I met Drew at the Middlesex. As his appointment was not until 1.30 he said he might as well go to work beforehand. His first task was to drink three cups of white gunk which contained the barium that would show up during the computer scan. It was two more hours before he was slid into the machine. I walked what seemed like miles to 'Snax', a cafeteria on the ground floor, where I bought a cappuccino and an orange muffin made by Mrs Otis Spunkmeyer. I ate it in the corridor outside the scanner and read a newspaper.

Drew was distressed when he came out. It had finally dawned on him what he was facing. He broke down on the stairs. I hugged him, tried to reassure him, and fought back my own tears. I, too, felt like sinking to the floor and crying my eyes out – but not here, not in public. I had to be strong. I cajoled him outside into a taxi. When we got home he said he was going for a lie-down. 'Why don't you come too?' I lay beside him. Sleep, to my surprise, was the last thing on his mind.

That evening we had dinner with Geoff and Mandy at the Groucho. Martin Amis and Ian McEwan were at the next table. The superstar novelists were in the same room yet the gulf between us was so great, they might as well have been on a different planet. Drew enjoyed his duck confit, sea bass and pecan pie. Once again it was only when he went to the lavatory that I started to cry: 'I'm not strong enough. I can't do this.' 'You can,' said Mandy. 'You wanted to pay him back for all the things he's done for you. Now's your chance.' The candles on each table were reflected in the glass roof of the dining room. I was grateful that it was dark. When Drew returned I held his hand.

It was bound to happen sooner or later. The pressure that had been building up inside me had to be released. There is a huge difference between knowing how to behave and actually being able to do so. It was impossible to carry on as normal because normality had ceased to exist: we were going through an extraordinary time.

I should have cancelled the dinner party but Drew was looking forward to seeing Peter and Derek again. I invited Alex as well for moral support. He said very little when I told him Drew had cancer. Peter and Derek were kept in the dark. By Friday evening I was exhausted: everything – the shopping, the cleaning, the chocolate mousse – had taken so much more effort than usual.

Alex, who worked in public relations, and Derek, who had recently finished a run at the National, were at each other's throats from the start. Theatre and PR both involved putting on a performance but Alex responded to Derek's sniping at his industry by saying it was a bloody good thing that actors were now being forced to do other jobs instead of 'resting' on the dole. 'You'll learn more about life from emptying people's dustbins than poncing about on a stage.' Peter and Drew hardly spoke. No matter how much I drank I could not get drunk.

After dinner Alex demanded that we all play a game. Derek rejected Trivial Pursuit – too boring. Pictionary was too childish. Deprivation did not make sense. Truth or Dare, on the other hand, sounded interesting. However, when he would not answer his Truth question ('When were you last unfaithful to Peter?') or perform a Dare instead I decided it was time for him to go home. He refused to leave. I saw red. I turned off the music and began to clear away. Alex tried to calm me down but I was adamant. These fat queens did not matter. They were history. I picked up a kitchen knife. Would they please just get the fuck out?

Drew was very upset. I had let him down, I had let myself down, but I was too furious to care. I was just as furious the next day when Drew told me he had called Peter and Derek to apologise. Alex advised me to ask my doctor for some Diazepam. He never saw Drew again.

A ball came over the wall into the garden. We went down to retrieve it. The familiar chorus rang out: 'Thank you!' Spring had made the plants shoot up. The bare, brown plot had achieved a rank luxuriance. Drew had spent a couple of Saturday mornings digging around – he had unearthed the iris bulbs that now sat in pots on the terrace – but neither of us had found the time to hack back the undergrowth or even discuss what we should eventually do with our own green space. The garden was like our relationship: it had a great future behind it.

The lump on Drew's neck got bigger. He bit his nails down to the quick. I found myself recording every last detail about him: the way he always started reading a magazine from the back; the way he would suddenly scratch the side of his head in a spasm of perplexity; the way he left mugs right on the edge of the worktop. I was convinced they would fall off. He tried to talk to me about what I would do after he was gone. It just made me cry. I could not think about it. There could be no afterwards. I wished yet again that it had been the other way round. Drew would not have been alone for long.

I pressed on with *Snow Hill* and did not shut down the computer even if Drew arrived home from work: another source of guilt. I should have been spending every available second with him. I posted off the finished treatment to Carole Blake with a sense of relief not achievement. It was in someone else's hands now. That evening, when I kissed Drew goodnight and felt the warmth of his cheek, the thought sprang into my mind that one day it would be cold. I slept badly. The nightmare returned for the first time in months. I woke, drenched in cold sweat, convinced there was someone in my room. A light glowed under Drew's door. He was playing a game on the Amiga. He was due to hear the results of the CT scan in six hours.

*

We only had to wait an hour beyond the allotted appointment time. Dr Duchesne, the consultant, was unavailable so Dr Bloomfield, the registrar, saw Drew instead. 'Come with me,' said Drew. The quiet, ginger-haired man hardly looked old enough to be a doctor and yet he somehow found the strength to deal with the terminally ill every day. Not all the results had come in but the good news was that no other tumours had been detected. The bad news was that the tumour in Drew's groin was eight centimetres long, the size of an orange.

It was inoperable. The pelvic region was the only place that such a tumour could have grown without being noticed earlier. It must have been there for quite some time. They had not been able to identify the primary source of the melanoma. This was not important: they had to concentrate on the areas to which it had spread. The best way to combat the tumours in his groin and neck was a course of chemotherapy.

We were in the hot, bright office for over an hour. Drew asked lots of questions, Dr Bloomfield answered them all and I listened. How much pain would there be? Would he be able to travel, to sit at a desk? Would he turn into a vegetable? Were there any useful books he could read? How about meditation or alternative medicine? Were there any experimental cure programmes he could join? Would further exposure to the sun speed up the spread of the cancer? Could he still drink alcohol? Would he be able to donate any parts of his body or would they all be corrupted? Would it all end quickly or slowly?

Drew left the consulting room with a sheaf of prescriptions. It took more than half an hour for the pharmacist to fill them out, by which time Drew was in pain. We left the main hospital building and set off for John Astor House, where the chemotherapy unit was based. We got lost and lost our tempers, bickering in Candover Street while office workers, their shirt sleeves rolled up, strolled to the sandwich bar in the sun. I felt utterly wretched and inadequate. I told Drew to wait where he was and hurried back to the oncology department. Jessica drew a map for me: we had been given the wrong directions.

It was cooler in John Astor House. After a brief introduction we were given a tour of the first floor along with another patient, a charming, middle-aged woman. I tried not to feel sorry for her: I had to save all my sympathy for Drew. The department was a place of subtext, of unspoken emotion. Pity lurked behind the smiles of the staff. The expressions glimpsed on the patients' faces ranged from barely suppressed panic to resignation and regret. They knew what we had coming.

We ate in a fish restaurant in Charlotte Street. Drew expected to start his treatment on the Monday. I explained that the second of May was a bank holiday. His days may have been numbered but other people still had to have their days off. Yes, it was a ludicrous system. Cancer did not recognise the calendar. Drew was worried that his hair would fall out. Dr Bloomfield had said this was unlikely but, whatever happened, I was determined Drew would not be reduced to wearing a baseball cap. Whether the headgear celebrated the New York Yankees or Tweety-Pie, the symbol of healthy, outdoor sports always made balding chemo patients appear pathetically jaunty.

When the 400mg of Ibuprofen had finally taken effect we walked down Tottenham Court Road, past *Time Out*, and round the corner into New Oxford Street. We had decided to go on a second P&O cruise. Drew should at least see Sydney before it was too late. We booked the best possible cabin on a ship that set sail from Hong Kong in December and arrived in Sydney Harbour on New Year's Day. I had no idea how we were going to pay the £8,000 fare: if it came to it I would cash in my life assurance. Drew did not have such a policy or a pension – he had suggested insuring his life before Christmas but there had seemed no cause to hurry – another reason why it would have been better if I had become ill instead. The last time I was in this office I had been booking my berth on the Caribbean cruise. Sixteen months had passed: now Drew was going home to die. At least he would do it in style. If it had not been for me he would have returned to Australia straight away. They had more experience of fighting skin cancer down under.

The Forbidden Planet bookshop was next door. Drew bought his favourite science fiction quintet. He wanted to read it yet again. Deprived of a future, he was already reliving, retreating into, the past. We spent the evening on the sofa, ordered Chinese, and talked about his tumour, which Drew had christened Lumpy. He must have had it when he met me. It had been between us all the time. The fact that it was in his groin, the centre of genital attraction, was a sick joke, an apparent reproach for what some would call our misguided lust. Drew nibbled my arm and announced he was a fruit bat.

The Middlesex Hospital called the following morning. Although it was Saturday Drew was required to register because his chemotherapy was to begin on the Tuesday. The drug would be administered to him as an in-patient since it was his first time. I could not go with him: I had too much work to do. Sally was ill and unable to do her television previews for the *Sunday Times*. My deadline was Monday: bank holidays meant nothing to newspapers.

Drew returned with Travel Scrabble from Hamley's and a pale blue plastic folder from the Middlesex. The cover was emblazoned with the teaching hospital's emblem and motto: '*Miseris Succurrere Disco*'. I learn to help the suffering. The information inside aimed to answer any questions a patient starting chemotherapy might ask:

> The chemotherapy you will be receiving is called DACARBAZINE (DTIC). This drug is given every three weeks, either as a single dose, or every day for five consecutive days. It is given as an infusion, into a vein in your arm and usually lasts approximately one hour. This treatment may be given either as an in-patient or as an outpatient.

The list of side-effects went on for pages: anaemia, nausea and vomiting, diarrhoea, constipation, venous pain, fever, facial flushing, restlessness and agitation. There was even a page about sex:

> Your illness and cancer treatment affect every part of your life, therefore it is not surprising that many patients find their sexuality is affected. This can manifest itself in many ways and may hardly bother you at all, but it can be a big problem. You may feel less whole while you are ill. Your role whether as bread-winner, home-maker or a combination of these may alter since you have to spend time having treatment away from home and work.

I was not a patient yet I had to force myself to read on:

> In spite of all the things that are happening to you, the changes that may be taking place in your body as well as your lifestyle, you still need affection. Cuddling and touching can be very reassuring and can help to make you feel loved and valuable.

The booklet concluded with offers of counselling. The tone was matter-of-fact, the outlook positive, but there was no way of getting round it: this was a guidebook to hell.

Drew's fear grew throughout the holiday weekend. He tried to work on the adventure novel he was writing for teenagers but soon gave up. He slept badly in spite of the tranquillisers. The world carried on just the same. The Republic of Ireland won the Eurovision Song Contest for the third time. Stephen Hendry beat Jimmy White in the final of the Embassy World Snooker Championship yet again. Once my copy had disappeared on a bike to the *Sunday Times* I settled down to do the Azed crossword. The word to be clued in this month's competition was 'mayday'.

8

FRESH HELLS

Drew cried his heart out before we left for the Middlesex. There was nothing I could do except hold him. I had to bully him out of the door: 'Come on. These people want to help you. It's for your own good. The sooner the drugs get to work, the sooner Lumpy will go.' That was the idea anyway.

The Prince Francis Ward was on the second floor. Newcomers were put in one of two private rooms to help them become accustomed to hospital life. My heart sank as we ran the gauntlet of beds that lined the walls. Every one was filled with a cancer patient: old, young, male, female, robust, wizened. I could feel their eyes follow us down the aisle. It was a relief when the door swung shut.

The hot, dark room felt like an airing cupboard. The bed took up most of the space. An adjustable table, a storage unit, an armchair covered in orange vinyl and a hard, straight-backed seat fought for the rest. A television, thank God, was fixed to the wall. There was a tiny, *en suite* bathroom containing a lavatory, wash-basin and shower. The only window looked out through pigeon-netting on to a dank lightwell. The view featured drainpipes, air-conditioning fans and more dirty windows. You could see a square of sky if you craned your neck. Still, anything was better than being out on the ward.

We played Scrabble, we watched television, we met most of the staff. It was not until 3.30pm that the Dacarbazine arrived in a sinister black bag. Sunlight rendered it ineffective. There was no danger of that in here. The needle – grimace – was inserted into Drew's left arm; the bag hung up on its drip-stand; and the electronic pump switched on. Red digits glowed in the gloom. The £1,000 worth of poison started to seep into his veins.

I did not want to leave him but everything seemed to be working and Drew assured me that he was okay. I promised I would return very soon. I checked the coast was clear then kissed him goodbye. I walked out of the ward, eyes fixed straight ahead, down the stairs, along the corridor, past the chapel and out into Mortimer Street. The daylight made me flinch.

We had not been missed. Life in the capital had continued as usual. The streets were clogged with workers, tourists and shoppers. Taxis made U-turns, buses ignored red lights, cyclists rode on the pavements. I made my way to Heddon Street, trudged up the stone steps to the top of Number 35 and told Panoptic the bad news. They had some for me as well: a second series of *Bad Ideas of the Twentieth Century* had been commissioned but I would not be needed on the first programme, 'Media-ism'. The presenter, Norman Stone, Professor of Modern History at Oxford, had his own researcher. At least I would be able to spend more time with Drew. I was back in his room by 5pm with a selection of treats from M&S.

The infusion had been successfully accomplished. I prayed that it would not make him sick. Drew was now on morphine as well. It made him sleepy but controlled the pain. Mandy called in for a couple of hours during the evening. When she left I joined Drew on the bed, lay back against his pillows and put my arm round his shoulders. This time I did not remove it when someone came in. Winnie was one of the older nurses. She looked but said nothing.

At 10.45 Drew said he wanted to go to sleep. I had been dreading this moment. He started to cry as I prepared to leave. I had to go: I could not spend every night in the armchair. I would go mad from lack of sleep. I reassured him I would be back tomorrow.

I was beside myself in the back of the cab as it rattled up Pentonville Road. How could I have been so stupid? Drew had found the lump in October. He had not seen a specialist until April, six months later. How could I have been so complacent? I should have taken more notice, insisted on a second opinion. All that time the tumour had been growing and we had done nothing about it. *Tempus edax rerum*. Cancer ate everything too.

*

Drew was supposed to be in hospital for five days but in the end he was in for ten. The Dacarbazine almost wiped him out. The pain in his side worsened. He spent the second night in the armchair because it seemed to hurt more if he lay down flat: 'Lumpy knows we're trying to kill him.' The morphine dose was increased so much that Drew's bowels soon turned to concrete. He took a viscous yellow solution called Co-danthramer to counteract the constipation. We nicknamed it 'Peach Juice'. Suppositories had no effect either. He hardly noticed Geoff and Mandy when they came to see him. We shared the bottle of wine they had brought. I was grateful for their company. It was almost midnight when I kissed Drew goodnight.

He started vomiting as soon as I left. He did not sleep. I was shocked at the state he was in when I returned on Thursday morning. He threw up when his chemotherapy began after lunch and when his dinner arrived at six. Dr Bloomfield told him that he should start a course of radio-therapy as well and stay in hospital over the weekend. Drew burst into tears. I nearly did too. I felt so impotent. We had lost control of our lives and those who did have control of them just seemed to be making matters worse.

More friends came to visit. Drew was a charming host but the effort exhausted him. Fiona, his boss at Thames Water, arrived later that evening, bearing flowers. I left them for a while and chatted briefly to Jenny, who had already become Drew's favourite nurse. 'We sometimes spend as much time looking after the relatives as the patients,' she told me. Then, seeing my guilt-stricken face, she added: 'Not you, silly. I've seen the way you two are together. You're wonderful.' I started to cry. Kindness was almost as difficult to deal with as the distress.

I promised Drew that I would be with him by ten o'clock on Friday morning. I bought my ready-to-eat lunch and dinner at M&S on the way in as usual and arrived half an hour early – even so, a porter was already wheeling him out of the ward. I followed them down to the radiotherapy department where Drew was measured, the target was set, and the tumour was zapped. Surely burning and poisoning would destroy it?

Drew was back in his cell by 11.30. He could hardly keep his eyes open. He threw up before his fourth dose of Dacarbazine but managed to keep down what little he ate of his dinner. He was put on a drip to rehydrate him. If he tried to talk he developed hiccups. The pain had gone and taken Drew with it. He had become a zombie in less than a week. Alison came at lunchtime with a big bunch of lilacs from her garden; Geoff and Mandy looked in at dusk. I felt even more isolated and alone when they had gone.

The weekend dragged. I was going to go to the gym on Saturday – I had not been since Monday; my shoulders ached – but Drew asked me to come straight to the Middlesex. I was there from ten till ten. Drew had his fifth and final dose of Dacarbazine and, apart from the odd bout of hiccups, felt as well as could be expected. I did not. The headache that I had woken up with mushroomed into a full-blown migraine. I was half-blinded by the aura when Howard and Sarah turned up in the afternoon with a clinking carrier-bag. I washed down four Migraleve tablets with the wine and became quite woozy. So did Howard: he pulled the emergency cord in the bathroom instead of the light-switch. It took ages to silence the alarm. Mandy popped in for an hour with another bottle of wine. Drew was so drugged up to the eyeballs he hardly knew we were there. He was a ghost at the feast. It was more difficult to be strong when he was not awake.

On Sunday, before I left for the hospital, I called Drew's parents. He was afraid that they would turn up on our doorstep. So was I. They seemed to believe me when I reassured them that the first week of treatment had gone well. Indeed, Drew was in much better shape when I saw him. He had been taken off the drip. We played Scrabble, watched TV, and even went for a walk down to the foyer. It was a sunny day; no one came to visit. The morphine, though, still made Drew dopey. I read the papers each time he dropped off. His parents rang in the evening. He was too weak to put on much of a performance, and they ended up upsetting each other. He was their youngest son and they wanted to be with him. 'I'll be home soon for good,' said Drew. 'When the chemo and radio have done their stuff I'm coming back to Australia.' He did not mention the cruise.

I tried not to think about the future. What would I do for money? Where would I stay? Drew's family did not know he was gay. They would not want me around, especially when they found out. Too bad. Where Drew went, I went. Till death do us part.

It was after eleven when I got home. I just wanted to go to bed but made myself sit at the kitchen table and apply for a job at the *Sunday Times*. I was shaking so much I could hardly write.

The mornings were the worst. I had to steel myself each time I entered the gloom of the entrance hall. I was leaving the world of work, health and play behind. It would be dark when I rejoined it – and Drew would be one day closer to his death.

On Monday Drew started to have anti-sickness injections in his backside. He still threw up. On Tuesday his temperature shot up to 39.5 degrees centigrade. He was put on an antibiotic drip. Chemotherapy made the patient susceptible to infection: it attacked the immune system as well as the cancer. His sheets had to be changed three times. He asked me to postpone all prospective visitors. The mobile shop, an overladen trolley, came round. A white-haired woman called Joan wondered if Drew would care for a manicure.

On Wednesday he rallied. It had been a good night. He had slept well, had not thrown up and had not even had the squits: diarrhoea was another side-effect. At least he could lay off the Peach Juice for a while. Dr Bloomfield said that his high temperature might be due to the tumour starting to break down. Drew's morphine intake had been halved, yet still he felt no pain. If there were no complications he should be able to go home the next day. It was wonderful to see the smile on his face. However, I was apprehensive at the prospect of having to care for him by myself.

Dr Duchesne resembled a young Maggie Smith. The consultant and her entourage arrived in Drew's room at 3.30 on

Thursday afternoon. Her charisma was not something she put on along with her white coat. It was clear she was liked as well as respected. After lunch an air of expectancy had filled the ward. The head girl was due. The staff acquired a spring in their step. The patients sat up. Each one hoped that she would be able to give them at least a crumb of comfort.

Drew examined Dr Duchesne as much as she examined him. She did her best to answer all his questions. He felt pain if he crouched down but otherwise the lower dose of morphine still seemed to be working. A metastatic malignant melanoma was a fearsome enemy: it could attack anywhere at anytime. It was a question of treating each symptom when and where it occurred. If things took a turn for the worse he could always come back to the ward.

Finally, after one last blood test, we left the Prince Francis at 4.45. I carried Drew's bags; he carried his drugs. The list of them filled all the space on his discharge sheet. It was a chemical arsenal: Co-proxamol, Voltarol, Sevredol, Cyclizine, Tamoxifen, Dexamethasone, Metoclopramide, Temazepam, Co-danthramer, Corsodyl, Difflam and Nystatin. There were pain-killers, anti-sickness pills, sleeping tablets, the familiar yellow laxative and mouthwashes. Mouth ulcers were just one more downside to the therapy. The various ingredients of the cocktail were meant to complement – and counteract the side-effects of – each other. As Dr Duchesne had implied, treating the tumour meant suffering one damn thing after another.

We returned to the Middlesex the next morning: Drew still required radiotherapy. We were home again by 8.30am.

Cabs were expensive but there was no alternative. We had been warned that the free hospital transport was erratic and time-consuming and there was no way Drew was fit enough to endure the discomfort of a bus ride. I was already sick of the to-ing and fro-ing. It was Friday the 13th. Drew was pale and gaunt, haunted. We were both exhausted and depressed. I did my best to raise his spirits, but it was not long before I knew I had failed.

We spent the weekend watching old movies: *Rebecca*, *The Little Foxes*, *All About Eve*. Drew rested or played his mindless computer games – until hot flashes down his left leg made him stop. He switched to the Game Boy that Geoff had lent him. Sunday was the first anniversary of our move into Packington Street, but neither of us felt like celebrating.

Drew was stretched out on the sofa beneath the linocuts. Their lines echoed in my head: 'The trees are coming into leaf like something almost being said . . . Their greenness is a kind of grief.' The white cherry blossom outside the window seemed to glow in the lingering light.

'I don't think I can go through all that again.' Drew turned to look at me. 'At least I could go to work before the chemo started.'

'Don't worry about work. The agency's giving you sick pay.'

'Only for twelve weeks.'

'It will all be over in two months. You've got two more courses to go. That's only two more weeks.'

'That's easy enough for you to say. You have no idea how awful it is.'

'I try, Drew.'

'I know you do. I'm sorry. I don't know what I'd do without you.'

'Go back to Oz.' Drew said nothing. A car with a boom-box in the boot shattered the silence. I hoped the bastard crashed.

'Have you asked about getting a visa?' he said finally.

'Not yet. There's no hurry.'

'We could still go on the cruise if we were already in Australia.'

'Do you want to go home sooner?'

'Sweetie, I am home. I'm with you. Does it matter where we are as long as we're together?'

'No. What would we do for money though? I wouldn't be able to work in Australia. Well, I could wash dishes I suppose.'

'My family would look after us.'

'You sure about that? It wouldn't take them long to find out. I wouldn't be so welcome then.'

'We could stay with my brother in Brisbane. I used to live with him.'

'And how would he feel about having two arse-bandits under his roof?'

'He'd be pretty cool, I think. He's an old hippie underneath.' I went over to him and sat on the arm of the sofa. I ruffled his hair. It was not falling out.

'You don't have to continue the treatment if you don't want to. It's entirely up to you. All I would say is that they wouldn't be spending thousands and thousands of pounds on you if they thought it was a waste of time. What's two more weeks of hell if it gives us longer together?'

'I don't like needles.'

'Neither do I. If they could stick them in me instead of you, believe me, I'd let them.'

'I know you would.' He took my hand. 'I don't want to lose you.' The lump in my throat was back almost immediately. It was never far away nowadays.

'You are not going to lose me, Possum. Just try. I'm not going to do a runner.'

'Jenny said that some partners walk out.'

'She told me that too. She was letting you know how lucky you are!'

'Some luck. I know what you mean though. I might not show it, but I am grateful.'

'You don't have to be. Just keep fighting, that's all I ask. You've been brilliant so far. You've been much braver than I would have been. I'm here because there's nowhere else I want to be.' I gave him a hug, making sure I rested my chin on his right shoulder. The lump on his left was bigger than ever. This is hell nor am I out of it.

'You know you always say I can ask you anything?'

'Yes.'

'Well, promise me that if things get really bad you'll help me end it all.'

'And how will you do that?'

'I don't know. Take all my pills. Jump off the roof. Listen to every REM CD. I don't want to turn into a vegetable. The

thought of being in pain and unable to move gives me nightmares. Promise me, Mark.'

'I promise. Now d'you want a glass of champagne or not?'
The subject made me uncomfortable. I was sure that if I had
been in his position I would have felt the same way. But it
would not come to that: Drew was just reassuring himself. I
put the idea out of my mind.

Early each morning the following week Drew received a dose
of radiotherapy. We fell into a cruel routine in which he woke
feeling better and came home feeling worse. I hated to watch
him limping down the zigzag ramp into the treatment room.
It had to be underground to protect the healthy from the
emissions of the giant death-ray machine. The headaches and
nausea peaked in the afternoons. Drew rested while I revised
my own treatment. Carole had suggested where I might
improve *Snow Hill*.

'Get Well Soon' cards arrived almost every day. 'I hear
you haven't been feeling yourself lately . . .' said the one from
Thames Water, signed by thirty-four of his colleagues. 'At
least the Doctor cured you of something!' Drew put them up
in his bedroom at first but took them all down when he ran
out of space: 'They won't let me forget.'

At the end of the week, after his final session, Drew was
seen by a doctor and another blood sample was taken. They
were bleeding him dry. He was due to start his second
course of chemotherapy on the Monday. It was true he could
move more easily now, but his leg was numb. The doctor

pointed out that at one stage he had been on 200mg of morphine: today he was on just 30. The treatment must be working. I went shopping in the afternoon. When I got back Drew was eating a bowl of canned apricots and a plate of tomato ketchup. His tastebuds had gone haywire. There was an air of defiance about the way he spooned the slop into his mouth. He sometimes resented the fact that he had to rely on me so heavily. He reasserted his independence however he could.

He had planned to go to a cricket match with one of his colleagues on Sunday. I was relieved when it was rained off – the thought of him throwing up in a crowd of flannelled fools had been worrying me ever since he had announced his intention. The cancellation of his day out sent him into a sulk. He refused to come with me to Camberwell to visit Mandy, who was laid up with a bad back. I did not like leaving Drew by himself, but I also wondered if I was being over-protective. Mandy suggested Drew's parents use her flat when their impending visit could no longer be put off. She would stay with a friend. Drew seemed pleased that at least one problem had been sorted out, but I could tell the prospect of starting chemotherapy again was preying on his mind.

Drew did not want to go. He stood in the hall, exhausted, aching, weeping. I was not going to force him this time. 'It's up to you, Possum. Nobody else can make the decision.' We had a cuddle. He opened the door.

We arrived at John Astor House on time at 9.15am. At

10.15 a doctor came into the waiting room. Leo, the Senior House Officer, told Drew that his white blood-cell count was down to 55 – too low for chemotherapy. Drew immediately cheered up. Leo discussed Drew's case with him and explained that his bad dreams were probably caused by the anti-sickness steroid. As it would be another seven days before he started the second course of Dacarbazine it was safe for him to stop taking the drug. Drew smiled again. Leo had black, curly hair and white teeth. His white coat set off his Mediterranean tan to perfection. He looked more like an actor in a medical drama than a real doctor.

Drew's limp had become permanent. Surely this meant the tumour was growing not going? There was no way I could ask such a question in front of Drew. He said he could manage the walk to Gower Street, where I had to drop off the revised treatment of *Snow Hill* at my agent's office. Carole came out to meet us. 'This is the lady who is going to solve all our problems, Drew.' It was a stupid remark. The fact that Carole knew Drew was ill would not make it any easier for her to sell the book.

'I hope I can help,' said Carole, 'but I can't work miracles.' That did not bother me. I no longer believed in them.

Our friends rallied round. Drew could have had visitors every day if he had wished. Mandy and Henry were frequent callers; Alex and Geoff, however, were conspicuous by their absence. They restricted their calls to the telephone. They were busy, they were thinking of us, and I appreciated that. However, their new-found reluctance to come round to Packington Street made me think they were afraid that Drew's cancer was in some way contagious.

If Drew noticed their physical disappearance from our lives he did not say anything. His week-long reprieve was ruined by a fever. I had to change his sheets every day. The washing machine was on virtually all the time. Grey skies increased our sense of confinement. We watched old movies or argued over Scrabble. Drew snoozed fitfully or played with the Game Boy. I went to the gym a couple of times and worked my way through Robert Graves's *The Long Weekend*.

Drew veered between irritability and apathy. His mood darkened as each day passed. On Saturday evening Channel 4 celebrated the opening of the new Glyndebourne Theatre with a live, five-hour relay of the inaugural production, *The Marriage of Figaro*. I drank a bottle of fizz; Drew, a bottle of elderflower pressé. I cooked sirloin steak: perhaps the meat would build him up.

He burst into tears when I got into his bed. It had been a long time since he had let me touch him. The radiotherapy made him sore. Artificial sun-burn to cure skin cancer had never seemed like a good idea. His hair had begun to thin. I held him till the sobs subsided. I was warm, drowsy and depressed. It was good to feel his bottom in my lap again.

'Uh-oh.' Drew reached round and gripped my erection. 'What d'you expect me to do with this?'

'Whatever you want.'

'I'm not in the mood.' He turned over and threw the duvet

back. He was not hard. 'If you do something for me though I'll do something for you.'

'And what's that?'

'Kiss Lumpy. He's part of me – and if you love me then you must love him.' I could not love the lump. I hated it. There were times when I felt like plunging my hand into Drew's groin and ripping the evil fungus out. It was a sickening request. The Drew I knew would not have made it.

'Go on. Prove your love for me.' I lowered my head, closed my eyes and touched it with my lips. 'Thank you.' I lay back.

'Oh dear.' He laughed. I had gone limp.

Monday 30 May was another bank holiday, another delay of twenty-four hours. I spent the afternoon cancelling the French trip that we had planned for September and filling in an insurance claim to recoup the deposit.

Drew had to have a blood test before the chemotherapy could be resumed. We walked from the lab round the corner to John Astor House. Half an hour later Leo told us that, although Drew's white blood-cell count had returned to normal, his haemoglobin levels had dropped. He needed to have a blood transfusion before he could receive any further treatment. The future looked very bleak. If one course of chemotherapy had almost annihilated Drew, what would he be like after three? We trailed back to the blood labs for a second test so that the transfusion could be cross-matched; traipsed to the X-ray department so that his lungs could be checked; and queued in the pharmacy for yet another bottle of Peach Juice. In the meantime Drew chewed his way through a whole packet of wine gums and then demanded a Magnum. His constant craving for ice-cream marked a further retreat into childhood.

The transfusion took place on the following Thursday in John Astor House. Each patient had their own room in the chemotherapy suite. Drew sat in an armchair and gazed at the plane trees outside. Their threshing leaves appeared to be trying to clean the window. He was given three pints of blood over six hours. He only threw up once. An Australian chaplain looked in and, having enjoyed a good lunch, stayed to give us the story of his life. He camped it up, he swore, but he talked a lot of sense. When he asked me what I did I said I was a writer. I usually said that I was a journalist. The word sounded wrong.

The next morning I received the punishment for my presumption: a letter from my agent rejecting *Snow Hill*. Was there a way I could 'inject more passion into it'? I was crushed. My hopes were dashed. I could not think any more. Despair would be the only emotion I could add to *Snow Hill*. It would have to be put on ice. I had betrayed Drew's faith in me.

The post contained more bad news. Drew had been fined £125 for speeding on 5 November and his driving licence would be endorsed. He did not seem concerned by either disappointment. No doubt such let-downs were insignificant when compared with the betrayal of his own body.

It was a horrible weekend. Drew resumed taking the Cyclizine and started vomiting more frequently. His right arm began to hurt too. I was in a foul mood, resentful of my defeat. I hated myself for snapping at Drew. I said things that I knew should not be said and yet this did not stop me. He lay on his bed reading or just stared at the stain on the ceiling. 'So that's it, is it? You're just going to lie there and rot for the rest of your life?' I pressed on with my chores but broke down as I scrubbed the bathroom sink. The last words Kenneth Williams wrote in his diary before committing suicide echoed in my mind: 'What's the bloody point?' In the end I joined Drew on his bed, his exhaustion merging with mine. When Caroline, one of his friends, arrived with her husband to go for a walk with Drew on Sunday afternoon, we did not answer the door.

I missed Drew even though he was still with me. The boy I met at the Barbican had already gone. I missed the support he gave me. My friends did their best but, for all their love and attention, they could not compensate for the intimacy I now felt to be lacking. Such selfish thoughts made me feel even more useless.

Drew finally began his second course of chemotherapy at 12.30pm on Monday 6 June. D (for Dacarbazine) Day. At 10.30 Dr Stephanie Gibbs gave him the results of his morning blood test and the go-ahead for another five-day dose of the toxic tonic. It was all over in sixty minutes. The insertion of the cannula, a tube supposed to facilitate hypodermic injections, was the greatest part of the ordeal.

I got out of the cab at the Angel to do some shopping.

When I got home Drew showed me a postcard of the Ashton Memorial. It was addressed to 'Drew'. My mother did not know his surname:

> I just thought I would send you a few postcards of Lancaster so that you can see what Mark and Howard may talk about sometimes. Regards, Brenda Sanderson

She was trying, bless her. This was a woman who had sent her son-in-law a birthday card asking, 'How do you catch gay mice?' The punchline inside sniggered: 'Use a poofy cat.' Perhaps she did know after all. My sister did because I had told her two days earlier on her twenty-eighth birthday. She had guessed as much. She too had sent a card to Drew.

> Just to let you know that I've been thinking of you. I'm glad I know how much you and Mark mean to each other. I thought you might be amused to see these photos of Mark when he was young! Take care, love, Linda xx

These gestures probably meant more to me than Drew. It was my fault that they amounted to a case of too little, too late. The prospect of losing him had loosened my tongue. It was an example of past cowardice, not present bravery. My family would never get to know Drew now. If they had seen how much I loved him surely they would eventually have loved him too?

We returned to John Astor House at 10am the next day.

There had been some kind of mix-up with Drew's prescription so we had to wait three hours for the drug to arrive. And Drew's cannula had to be replaced first. It was supposed to last for several days. Drew was buoyed up by the fact that he only required 10mg of morphine that day but it proved too great a reduction. The tumour soon woke up. He was back on 30mg on Wednesday. The Dexamethasone continued to give him nightmares so he was not given an injection of the anti-sickness steroid. However, having thrown up at 7pm, he reluctantly took a Dexamethasone pill. He was caught between the devil and the deep blue bucket.

On Friday morning I woke to the sound of Drew vomiting. Two milligrams of Dexamethasone were not enough. He doubled the dose. His cannula had to be replaced for the third time that week before he could receive his fifth bag of Dacarbazine. Afterwards, Raj, the charge nurse, said they might put in a central line next time round: a butterfly valve inserted directly, and semi-permanently, into a vein in his chest.

Drew was weeping before we got through the front door. 'I'm sick of people sticking needles in me. I'm sick of throwing up. The tumours are still growing. I don't want to be in pain any more. This is not quality of life. I want to die. I want to die right now.' I tried to hold him but he shoved me away. 'Is that the best you can do? You promised you'd help.'

'Drew, it's too soon.' I was shocked. He was beginning to scare me. This was not just another panic attack. 'I will help you. Please don't ask me to keep my promise yet. You've got to help me too. What will I do without you?'

'Oh, for pity's sake. You'll find someone else.'

'I don't want anyone else. I've given all my love to you. You're everything to me. Without you I'm nothing.'

'Look, I know all this has been bad for you as well but I'm the one who's in pain, I'm the one who's dying. Now will you help me or not?'

There were a couple of letters on the carpet. I picked them up and opened them. It was an excuse not to say anything. I did not know what else to say. The first was a rejection from the *Sunday Times*. The second was from the claims department of American Express requesting a copy of Drew's death certificate. I sank to the floor, tears streaming down my face. I could not take any more.

'What is it?' I handed him the letters. I could not stop crying. Perhaps we should go upstairs and swallow all his tablets. There were enough to take half of Islington with us. After a while I felt Drew's hand on my shoulder. 'I'm sorry. I hate it when you cry. I'm a big selfish pig. Will you make me a cup of Horlicks? You do it better than me.'

As I stood in the kitchen waiting for the milk to boil I realised that things could only get worse. I already knew that if I were ever diagnosed with terminal cancer I would not have chemo or radiotherapy. Drew seemed determined to arrange his own death. I was glad that he felt he could ask me to help but at the same time wished he had not. What would I do if I were him? Would I leave him a note and then jump off Tower Bridge with a brick in each pocket? Surely the shock of that would be easier to deal with than helping me to kill myself? It was impossible to say. I would want to spend as much time with Drew as possible. I would want him to be with me at the end. Running away to die alone might be seen as an act of betrayal. Drew had not run off back to Australia, and I was not going to desert him.

We spent the following afternoon on the south bank of the Thames. Sun glinted off the river. A flotilla of wherries sailed past the National Theatre. We were there to see a matinée performance of *Pericles*:

> Oh you gods!
> Why do you make us love your goodly gifts,
> And snatch them straight away?

Drew had not mentioned suicide again. It was a dreadful production, more like a Music & Mime lesson at school than Shakespeare for grown-ups. Drew enjoyed it though. I was on tenterhooks: he could have thrown up at any moment. The side-effects of the chemotherapy had kicked in much earlier this time.

On Tuesday morning I heard a cry from Drew's bedroom. I ran upstairs to find him holding up one of the bookcases. It was about to topple over him. We forced it back against the wall but the weight of books had become too great. The frame returned to a slant no matter how many times I straightened it up. I lost my temper and started flinging the paperbacks off the shelves. Drew, who stood directly in the line of fire, retreated to the landing. Once I had started I just kept going. Soon only the bottom shelf had books on it: the volumes of Contemporary Literary Criticism were too heavy to throw around. We left the mess as it was and walked to the bank on Islington Green then sat in the sun till lunchtime. The collapse had been an omen. I had been worrying what to do with my library ever since it seemed we were going to Australia. A kind and helpful man at the High Commission had advised me to apply for an ordinary three-month tourist visa then apply for an extension on compassionate grounds while I was out there.

I could not take my library with me – I had no wish to watch it moulder in the tropical humidity of Cairns – and storing it in Britain would be expensive. The sensible option was to sell the collection. We needed the money. Losing the library would be nothing compared to losing Drew.

Two days later it was gone. Jay McInerney's *Bright Lights, Big City*, Martin Amis's *Money*, Bruce Chatwin's *The Songlines* with the author's own handwritten correction on page 277, went into the back of a dealer's car along with all the other signed and unsigned first editions, review copies and proofs. The collection of a lifetime had brought me less than two months' rent. I kept the reference books and, for sentimental reasons, about thirty others, including Thomas Pynchon's *Gravity's Rainbow* – one of the few novels to change the way I saw the world. The living room sounded strangely echoey now. The empty shelves symbolised our hopeless future.

Drew handed me the yellow, laminated card. 'Here, you might as well use this.' It was his gym membership card. 'I won't be needing it for a while.' I was due to start work again at Panoptic on 20 June. His gym would be far more convenient than mine. I did not wait till then to try it out. A single swipe of the card and I was through the turnstile. The pool was usually unoccupied in the middle of the afternoon. I ploughed up and down, gradually entering an aquamarine trance, letting the world fall away, thinking of nothing and no one. The reverie vanished as soon as I stopped.

Drew went to work on Friday 17 June: 'At least I'll have the weekend to recover.' I had to restrain myself from calling him every hour. He returned at 5.30pm, glad to have gone. He had clearly been made very welcome. On Sunday Howard and Sarah picked us up in their new red convertible and, with the top down, we drove to Aston Clinton in Buckinghamshire. We had a pub lunch and then played croquet in the garden. Drew was not up to it. He sat on a bench in the sun while a Harrier jump-jet from the local air show screamed overhead. I wanted to scream too. In less than two months Drew had become an old man. Ten minutes later he asked: 'Can we go home now?'

On Monday morning he got up to go to Reading but had to go straight back to bed. The constant headaches and nausea had left him exhausted. I had to leave him to go to work. I should have stayed with him, I wanted to stay with him: economic necessity was forcing us apart.

Drew felt much better the next day. A note on the kitchen table told me he would be at Thames Water if I needed to talk. However, at 1pm he called Panoptic to say he was leaving the office. He was in bed when I got home. 'I think I've got a tumour in my right leg.' We agreed that he must give up all thought of work until he had recovered from his third course of chemotherapy. Our options were becoming ever more stark: insolvency in Britain or dependency in Oz.

It was a struggle to concentrate at work. Should Matthew Parris, the presenter of 'PR-ism', be filmed wearing Calvin Klein underpants in a South Molton Street boutique? Did it really matter? I spent most of my time trying to arrange a tea-party for the public-relations representatives of Chanel, Gucci, Cartier, Tiffany, Ralph Lauren and Louis Vuitton. We nicknamed them the Bond Street bimbos. When I happened to pick up a telephone call to Michael from Jo, the former colleague I had holidayed with in France, I ended up telling her the whole sorry saga of Drew. Thus far we had told as few people as possible but I was finding it more and more difficult to hold back. Almost two years had passed since our stay at Le Lac and here I was, still out of my depth. Jo, as usual, said the right thing. 'You were alone then. You're with Drew now.'

We were, without doubt, enduring the worst period of our lives. However, it was about to get worse.

9

THE LONGEST DAY

We arrived in Dagmar Road at the same time as Drew's parents. Drew got out of the minicab, slowly, and limped over to their taxi. I hung back. I had expected to meet Jack and Aileen one day but in Cairns, not Camberwell. Drew made the introductions. His father had a very firm handshake.

Mandy was not ready. Ten minutes later she opened the front door and invited us all in for breakfast. Jack and I carried the suitcases. No one accepted the offer of champagne. I sat in the garden with my coffee and croissant and let the Morgans have some time alone.

When John, Mandy's friend and colleague, arrived, they loaded up her Golf with the luggage in the hall. Mandy gave Mr and Mrs Morgan a last-minute briefing about the flat, kissed Drew and I goodbye, then handed over the keys. At 10am we left the visitors to get some sleep and walked up to

Camberwell Green. The weird reunion was over. I already knew it was going to be a long three weeks.

Drew got out of the cab at the Elephant & Castle and took the Tube back to the Angel. I reluctantly went on to Panoptic. At 6pm Drew pushed open the heavy, white door into the office. I could see that the Heddonists were shocked by the change in him. After a glass of water we took a cab back to Camberwell – not to Dagmar Road but to the College of Art round the corner, where Mandy and Henry escorted us through the final degree shows in the departments of ceramics, graphics and animation. One student had designed no less than twenty tea-pots. Drew particularly liked the one in the shape of an octopus. Its beak formed the spout. We bought it.

Drew began to feel ill in the college bar. Mandy and John drove us home. I was starving and wanted to order a Chinese but Drew was not hungry. A minute later he said he was going to be sick. I fetched the bucket. His vomit was black.

'I've got a stitch in my left side.' He staggered over to the sofa and lay flat out. 'It's spreading. It's getting worse.' I gave him some Sevredol. It had no effect. The pain got worse still. He turned grey and started to breathe erratically.

I called the Middlesex Hospital. The phone rang and rang in the Prince Francis Ward. When it was eventually answered I was told in broken English that there were no beds. I recognised the voice: it belonged to the Spanish auxiliary who brought round the hot drinks trolley each evening. I asked for Leo: 'Not here.' I asked for Jenny: 'Not here.' In the end a nurse suggested that I call Drew's GP. I did so. None of the six doctors in the local practice was on call. Would I like a locum? I said yes but, as soon as I replaced the receiver I picked it up again and, for the first time in my life, dialled 999.

I was ready in two minutes. Drew was in agony. 'I never knew such pain existed,' he whispered. Then, 'I love you.' I was shaking, trying not to cry. I knelt down and held his hand.

'I love you, Drew. I will always love you.' We both thought it was the end.

The ambulance took thirty minutes to arrive. It was not as if we lived in the back of beyond. My naïve faith in the emergency service was shattered. Drew was in so much pain he could not bear to be touched. 'He thinks he's dying,' I said to the plump paramedic as she puffed up the stairs. 'And is he?' she replied. I explained the situation.

'We can take him to Bart's,' said the driver. 'Will that do?'

'Well, he can't stay here, can he?'

'I'll get the chair then.'

The paramedics gave Drew oxygen for his pain. It was useless. They refused to give him anything stronger. They insisted he get into the wheelchair.

'He's got a massive tumour in his groin. Can't you use a stretcher?'

'Not down them stairs.' It took Drew ages to sit in the chair. He was in total, utter agony.

The ambulance looked like it had seen action in the Second World War. Its cream paint was chipped; the red vinyl seats were cracked. The blue lights flashed but the siren remained silent. The woman tried to make conversation as we rattled along through the dusk. I ignored her and concentrated on Drew. Every jolt made him wince. Our route took us over eighteen speed bumps.

We waited outside on the pavement for the security door to be buzzed open. The Accident & Emergency department was a dump. The Conservative government was threatening to close down St Bartholomew's but faced fierce local opposition. In the meantime, though, no money was being spent on the hospital. Depression and defeat lurked in the warm, stale air.

A pair of nurses undressed Drew painfully and wired him up to an electrocardiograph. I explained that he needed morphine and lots of it. They said a doctor would be along shortly. It was chaos. A baby was screaming, a stinking tramp was shouting, drunken yahoos were singing. We could hear but not see what was going on. I was afraid one of the idiots would burst through the curtain at any moment. This was no place for sick people.

And all this time Drew was in agony. He refused to swear and restricted himself to muttering 'shivers'.

'Go on, Drew, say "shit". It'll make you feel better.' His strength of character was amazing.

After half an hour a doctor, dead on his feet, slipped into the cubicle. 'Mr Drew?' I explained the situation yet again. He had not got a clue.

'He needs morphine. He must have morphine now.' Another thirty minutes passed. Two thugs arrived to wheel Drew to the X-ray department. It had been decided to admit him. However, he could not simply be put to bed: he might be an emergency case but he still had to complete the admissions procedure. 'He's got terminal cancer. Why does he need an X-ray?'

'Don't ask us, mate.' I followed them through a succession of scarred swing doors and down empty corridors which seemed to double back on themselves. Drew had to sit up for the X-ray: more prolonged, unnecessary pain.

One of the porters sloped off while Drew was being photographed. I took the other end of the trolley. 'You can't do that,' said the tattooed man. 'The insurance . . .' The Cockney nurse who had accompanied Drew saw the look on my face. 'I'll do it. We'll be here all night otherwise.' And, when the porter began to complain, she snapped, 'Oh, shut your cakehole.'

We trundled back to Casualty where Drew was finally given a couple of painkillers. They lasted ten minutes. We waited and waited. The yelling and scuffling became more sporadic. By midnight I had had enough. If making a scene was the only way of getting attention then I would make one. I told Drew I would be back in a minute, swept back the curtain and marched over to the nurses' station.

A Sister tried to shush me but she soon shut up. My name was Mark Sanderson, I wrote for the *Sunday Times*, and if Drew Morgan was not seen by a real doctor in the next five minutes I would be on the phone to the Health Secretary first thing in the morning. I would not only demand an enquiry into the gross inefficiency and life-threatening incompetence of this department but would start a personal crusade in the pages of every newspaper to explain why this hell-hole should

be closed down forthwith. My boyfriend was dying of cancer.
He had been in agony for the past three hours. *Now would
someone please give him some fucking morphine?*

I only shouted the last sentence. I knew I looked ridiculous:
I had changed into tracksuit bottoms and a Hawaiian T-shirt as
soon as we had got home. In the ensuing panic I had slipped a
pair of loafers on to my bare feet. My eyes were bloodshot,
my face was unshaven, and my whole body was shaking. I did
not give a damn though. All I cared about was stopping
Drew's pain.

Five minutes later a medic appeared. 'Sorry about the
delay. It's been a bad night.' His pager started bleeping. He
examined Drew briefly then turned to the nurse. 'He needs
a morphine pump.'

'That's what I've been saying since we got here at nine
o'clock.'

'He'll soon be more comfortable.' The doctor gave me the
ghost of a smile and moved on.

It was after two when the Cockney angel and I pushed
Drew across the windswept courtyard to the east wing. A
few stars peeped out from behind the clouds. There was an
underground route but this was quicker. We took a complaining lift to the third floor. A couple of nurses were still
noisily clearing lumber from the side-room off Garrod Ward,
where Drew was to spend the night. All the beds in the large
square room were occupied. At least Drew would be by himself. The harrassed pair acted as if they were doing us a huge
favour. I would be doing them a favour when I helped shut
down this ugly, old-fashioned, dispiriting pile.

The Cockney nurse said goodbye and hurried back to Casualty. An Irish girl settled Drew down, checked his pump, and returned to the desk that sat in a pool of yellow lamplight in the ward. Drew opened his eyes. 'It's almost over.'

'Don't say that.'

'I mean today. It's been the longest day, even if the date is wrong.'

'I must tell your parents. Strange how this all happened as soon as they turned up. It's as if you were hanging on.'

'I'm still hanging on. Call them in the morning. Let them rest.' I wasn't sure he would last till the morning. 'You better get to bed as well.'

'I'm all right. I'll stay here.'

'No you won't. You look worse than I do. I feel much better now, honest. Come back in the morning.'

'We must let Leo know what's happened too. You can't stay here.'

'Anywhere's better than where we just came from. Go on, I'll be okay.'

'In a minute.' I was terrified that this would be our final farewell. I did not have the strength to face it. I sat down on an ancient chair. 'I just need a breather. I've been on my feet all night. It's all right for you . . .' I was beginning to babble.

'Mark, I am not going to die. Well, I am – but not tonight.'

I started to cry. 'I don't want to leave you.'

'You must, or you'll be no use to me tomorrow. I won't be able to sleep with you squirming on that seat. Go home!'

I kissed him goodbye – 'I love you so much' – made sure the nurse had our home telephone number, and ran down the steps to the courtyard. The fountain was not playing, St Bartholomew the Less was dark but, across the road, Smithfield was a cathedral of light. It had occurred to me while researching *Snow Hill* — the police station in the story was only a minute away — that the hospital and its neighbour the meat market had a lot in common: both were body shops, both dealt with corpses every day. I had even set one chapter in the mortuary at Bart's.

The ranks of refrigerated lorries hummed to themselves as I trudged beneath the clock in the market's central avenue — ten past three — and watched an empty cab disappear up St John Street. It began spitting with rain. There was a blister on my right heel. Was there any point in going on? For a moment I actually stopped and thought about it.

A taxi pulled up. Its light was off. There was an ad on the passenger door: '*Time Out*: London's Living Guide'.

'Where you headed, mate?'

'Islington. Packington Street.' It was only when I felt for my keys that I realised that I had left my wallet behind.

'Hop in. It's on my way home.'

'The thing is . . .' — I was going to regret this — 'I've no money on me. Can I pay you when I get there? It won't take me a minute to get the cash.'

'No problem.' Was I dreaming? If only all cabbies could be like him. We reached Packington Street in less than ten minutes. I kicked off my shoes and ran upstairs to fetch my wallet. When I got back to the front door the good Samaritan had vanished.

*

I woke at 8am on the dot. The telephone had not rung during the night. I called the Prince Francis Ward. Bart's had been on to them already: Drew would be transferred to the Middlesex that morning. I called Drew's parents and told his father the news. We both became upset. I was unable to speak when his mother came on the line.

I had a bath, collected a few of Drew's things, and caught a cab back to the hospital. It looked better in daylight. Drew had managed to get some sleep, and his pain was under control. I sat with him till half-past eleven, at which point his parents arrived along with the ambulance crew. There was no room for me in the back of the vehicle – my eyes met his mother's as its doors closed – but I was going to Heddon Street, not Mortimer Street.

I waited till after lunch to make the telephone call. I had decided that not knowing was worse than knowing. I was wrong. Leo told me that the cancer had spread to Drew's liver and kidneys. His life expectancy was therefore two months, not two years.

I exploded with grief. Mary and Jean gathered round to comfort me and were soon in tears too. His vomit was black because he was bleeding internally. He needed more tests to ascertain the full extent of the cancer.

He was in bed 13 which, despite its number, was the best in the open ward. It was situated in a corner alongside a bay-window which looked out on to Nassau Street. That was as close as we would ever get to the Bahamas again. Although it was almost 6pm, Drew was just being wheeled off to the X-ray department. He asked me to follow him. His parents stayed where they were. When the porter went whistling off Drew dropped his bombshells.

'I've told my parents about us. It's okay. We've had a good talk and they agree that the best thing for us to do is to go back to Australia as soon as possible.' I was shocked. It was all very well for him to say that it was okay, but his parents were not going to take out their anger, grief and disappointment on him. 'Don't worry. It'll be all right. Mum said you can stay with us. You should've seen her face though when she learned that I'd put you down as my next of kin.'

The weekend provided a respite of sorts. The test results would not be ready till Monday. Drew was very poorly but remained aware of what was going on. He studied the three of us as we sat, stood and snoozed by his bed. He was the centre of our universe. It was inevitable that our orbits would become more and more erratic.

Jack, born in 1924, was twelve years older than my own father. Drew had inherited his short, stocky frame but not his complexion. Jack's skin was tanned and corrugated, like crocodile hide. I now understood why his son had been afraid of ageing, had spent hours applying moisturisers, even used facial mud-packs once a month. The retired dentist knew everything about everything and would happily share his knowledge with anyone who would listen. His wife, however, had no time for his lectures. She devoted all her attention to Drew. Jack's deep, resonant tones heightened the fragility of Aileen's quavering voice. Her shoulders stooped under the burden of grief. She reminded me of some nocturnal animal, a vole perhaps, surprised by daylight. Even so, I could see she ruled the family.

Proof of this came late on Saturday afternoon when Drew's sister, Debbie, arrived with her husband Simon, and their children Adrian, fifteen, and Carly, thirteen. Debbie's resemblance to Drew was unnerving: she was four years older yet they could have been twins. Uncle Drew was very fond of his nephew and niece: I had often posted presents to them on his behalf. Adrian, blond and slender, was a heartbreaker in the making. His freckly sister had none of his shyness. They gathered round Drew's bed and chattered away. I left at seven o'clock, hopelessly outnumbered. I planned to have an early night but ten minutes after I got home Mandy turned up to cook me dinner. We ate on the candle-lit terrace as zigzagging bats chased their own evening meals overhead.

The next morning Alex gave me a lift to the Middlesex. I had not seen him since the disastrous dinner party in April. Before I got out of the car he told me he would come to Australia for Drew's funeral. I spent eight hours with Drew that Sunday. He, like the rest of us, was still in a state of shock. His family drifted in and out at various times. Debbie and Simon wanted to show Adrian and Carly the sights. After all, as far as the kids were concerned, they were on holiday. Time was running out, yet I caught myself wishing that the long day were over. Tragedy can be boring too.

The full extent of the tragedy was spelled out the next day.

Drew was in a dreadful state, in greater pain, unsure what was happening to him. When he was wheeled off for another CT scan Dr Gibbs, Leo and a couple of nurses – Rae from New Zealand and Lisa from Guildford – assembled round his bed. I could feel the eyes of the ward upon us so I suggested we went into the day-room: a joyless collection of orange chairs, tattered magazines, incomplete jigsaws and dying spider plants. Its windows stared into the same lightwell that had made Drew's private room so gloomy. Dr Gibbs explained that Drew was critically ill: he was still haemorrhaging internally. He needed to be given pints of blood because his haemoglobin levels were very low. If possible I should stay with him rather than go to work.

I broke down and made a total fool of myself. I thought he was about to die. Dr Gibbs put her arms round my heaving shoulders while everyone else looked on uncomfortably. They must have sat through this scene countless times before. I felt guilty for taking up their time. I called Panoptic to let them know that I would not be coming in and sat beside Drew's bed awaiting his return. His parents arrived. We spent the rest of the day watching the red-black blood drain into his veins.

The downward spiral tightened daily. On Tuesday I found Drew wearing an eyepatch. The lack of platelets in his blood had made him lose the sight in his right eye. Drew, for some unknown reason, had always feared being blinded in an acid attack. His every nightmare seemed to be coming true. When he was given a transfusion of platelets an abreaction to them caused a violent shaking fit. His stomach became distended. He threw up a couple of times and consequently gave up trying to eat. The massive doses of morphine were causing severe constipation but it was too dangerous to give him suppositories or an enema: he was still bleeding inside. And, after all this, when his parents had reluctantly left for Camberwell, I had to get Drew to sign some blank cheques so we could use his sick-pay to settle a few bills.

On Wednesday Drew had a bone-scan in the radio-clinical department. The porters came for him in the middle of his lunch and refused to wait. He was not eating much anyway. The huge scanner squatted in the centre of the chilly room. I watched Drew glide into its maw then went to wait outside. It looked right through him for twenty-five minutes yet found no trace of leukaemia. However, that did not mean his bone marrow was not affected. A sample would have to be taken. Early the next morning, with deep reservations, I gave the haematologist permission to proceed. Drew had endured another bad night. Lack of sleep had reduced his resilience to zero. He was a voodoo doll in never-ending pain. When he felt the needle puncture his skin he burst into tears. It was not the pain, he said, it was the whole scenario. He wailed unashamedly. The whole ward went quiet. The haematologist left us alone to weep together. Twenty minutes later he returned with a happy drug that was supposed to relax Drew for ten minutes. It knocked him out for two hours. The staff were so concerned they stopped the morphine pump. While Drew was unconscious, the haematologist skewered his pelvic bone – twice. The first attempt failed. At 4pm, I left him with his parents and went into Panoptic for a couple of hours. While I was away there was another crisis. Drew needed a second transfusion of platelets. It took four attempts to insert a new cannula. 'I want Mark, I want Mark,' cried Drew. No one called me. He was still receiving the platelets when I returned. A nurse told me what had happened. Why? Was she punishing me for my apparent desertion? Trying to hurt me with Drew's pain? I felt like punching her.

The fact that Drew and I were lovers was not mentioned at all. Jack would talk to me about shells, or golf, or garbage disposal, but not about anything that mattered. Aileen seemed to be constantly biting her tongue. I had kept my parents out of the mess for as long as I could – they had my grandmother to look after – but I had to talk to someone. That evening I called my father and explained our parlous financial situation. 'Well, I won't let you starve.' He suggested I file for bankruptcy until I pointed out that my assets – Shakespeare Walk, primarily – far outweighed my debts. He then said that I should move out of Packington Street as soon as Drew died. I already knew that I could not, would not, lose my lover and my home. I would lose my mind if I did. Drew and I had been at our happiest in Packington Street. If I quit the flat our entire relationship would seem like a dream. There would be nothing, apart from a few photos, to show that it had ever happened. These walls had witnessed everything. They would always contain our love.

I did not think this was the moment to tell my father that his son was queer. I had vaguely planned to tell my parents formally in a few years' time, when it would have been obvious that Drew and I were 'married'. Besides, the honourable way would be to break the news in person, not on the telephone. However, four hours later, I could contain myself no longer – Drew was dying, for Christ's sake – so I called my mother and poured my heart out to her.

Had she known her son was gay? 'I'd had my suspicions.' There was a hardness in her voice that I had not heard before. 'Whatever you do, don't tell your father.'

'Why not?'

'It'll kill him.' I was surprised by her certainty. I explained what Drew and I were going through, tried to sound positive and confident, but my mother seemed too shocked to offer much sympathy or understanding. 'It's such a shame that his parents had to find out.' I could not believe my ears.

'Would you rather I were dead than gay?'

'You know what I mean. If Drew hadn't told them it would have been one less thing for them to worry about.' My mother, of course, saw the crisis through their eyes, not ours. In other words, she wished I had not told her.

'How would you feel if Dad was dying of cancer? Well, that's exactly how I feel about Drew.'

I was glad that I had finally told my mother – and I was proud that Drew had given me the courage to do so – but my timing had been bad. Instead of improving the situation, my moment of weakness had made things worse for us both. There was now a distance between my mother and I and a secret between my parents.

*

July came in on a heatwave. I went for a swim at Drew's gym. The sheer health of the bodies on view was overpowering. There were no grey faces, jaundiced eyes or necrotising necks here. The flesh was firm and tanned, not saggy and mottled. Each boy had an unwitting, everyday beauty. The woman in the subscriptions department had been in tears when she transferred Drew's membership over to me. When you enrol at a gym you expect the membership to expire, not you.

Drew was sitting up against a mountain of pillows. I handed him an M&S carrier-bag containing grapes, plums and prunes. He was still constipated. He showed me two lumps on his chest that had come up overnight. He was like a mushroom bed. There were tumours in seven other sites besides his groin, shoulder, liver and kidneys. Dr Gibbs had told him it was unlikely that he would survive for two months.

The chemotherapy and radiotherapy had not prolonged his life, they had hastened his death – and made his remaining time a misery. Their spectacular failure was more of a shock because the media was forever trumpeting medical advances: new discoveries, new drugs, new treatments. 'Doctors announce cancer treatment breakthrough', 'Aids virus offers hope of remedy for cancer', 'Scientists hail dual cancer treatment': such headlines created a false sense of optimism. When it came down to it, the doctors were still in the Dark Ages. Three hundred years ago their fellow practitioners were recommending dog-shit as a cure for eye infections.

When Drew's parents turned up I walked down to Panoptic. Jean presented me with a cheque for the balance of my salary and said they would manage without me. I ought to be with Drew. We drank a couple of bottles of cheap champagne to toast my departure. My mother called while I was there. The fact that she did was more important than what she said.

Drew was now taking 150mg of morphine a day. He became confused, unsure whether he was awake or asleep: 'Is this real?' His look of disappointment was heart-breaking. The evenings were the best times. His parents insisted on using public transport so they left around 8pm. I watched the lights come on in the flats across the road; watched people cook their dinner and eat it in front of the TV; laugh on the telephone; water the windowbox; stroke their cat. They seemed blissfully unaware of their own good fortune. The few yards that separated them from the ward might as well have been miles. In the fortnight that we spent there some patients did not receive a single visitor.

Drew's moods changed by the minute. He was petulant, euphoric, angry and desperate. I liked it when he lost his temper with me: it showed the real him had not been entirely smothered by drugs. The West End was gearing itself up for another Friday night and here we were discussing death, death, death. He had been back in the Middlesex for a whole week now. He knew he would never see Australia again.

'You won't forget your promise, will you?' He had taken off the eye-patch. It made him itch.

'No, of course not.' There was no one around. 'It won't be easy in here.' The point of no return was rapidly approaching. I had no problem with mercy killing in theory – it was basic common sense: suffering had no meaning – but could I actually carry one out? There was still time for Drew to take an overdose. Perhaps I could bring all his pills in from home.

'Leo said that I might be able to go home if they can stabilise my condition. I don't want to die in here.' We held hands. I had run out of words. 'Will you bring me in some more boxers tomorrow? These are getting really daggy.'

I tried to organise a shift-system so that Drew was left alone as little as possible. I should have saved my breath. His parents arrived one hour after I did on Saturday morning: it felt to me like they were pleasing themselves, not Drew. The atmosphere between us curdled. Aileen became ever more querulous. She used feebleness to mask her fury. She acted as though I was planning to steal her baby. Jack carried on talking whether or not anyone listened. Drew was put on antibiotics to counteract a fever. His morphine dosage went up to 200mg. It caused spasms throughout his body. I went to buy him a vanilla milkshake from Burger King. When I got back he was dishing out computer games. Carly was puzzled: 'Why are you giving us our Christmas presents now?'

I woke up crying on Sunday morning. I arrived at the Middlesex at the same time as his parents. Drew sent them away. The pain was spreading, his left leg was swelling – even his genitals had become distorted: 'Everything inside me is going wrong. I hate to think what'll happen next.' He swung in and out of lucidity, micro-napping in a morphine haze. He thought he might be going mad. At one stage he sat rocking on his bed chanting: 'I'm a loony. I'm a loony.'

Debbie, Simon, Adrian and Carly came to say goodbye. Photos, tears, champagne in plastic cups. I left them to it and went home to watch Wimbledon: Goran Ivanisevic was playing Pete Sampras in the final. It was all over in three straight sets. On my return a nurse asked who had won. I had no idea. Drew had one mouthful of his dinner, turkey casserole, and threw up. The sudden movement caused severe pains in his chest. His morphine intake was boosted. When he had recovered I took him to have a bath. I played with the controls of the cradle, making Drew go up and down over the water, but he was in no mood for fun: 'Stop it, stop it, stop it!' His body was blotched and bloated. I had to turn off the turbo-jets. They hurt too much. He complained of a new pain as I towelled him, gingerly. Leo came to see us at half-past ten. It was probably Drew's liver. His morphine dosage was increased to 240mg. Jenny suggested we contact the palliative care team.

The following morning he lay sobbing on his bed. The bone-marrow sample showed that it had been affected by the chemotherapy, that the cancer had spread to his head. The lack of motor control in his right arm was attributed to a brain tumour. The end-game had started. My main aim was to get Drew home as soon as possible. The thought of him being stuck in the corner of that ward alone, longing but unable to die, was unbearable.

On Tuesday a doctor from the palliative care team spelled out the options. As he was doing so Jack and Aileen arrived. Drew sent them off to the day-room. Drew could either have an epidural which would eventually wear off or a coeliac block which would not. This involved destroying with drugs the nerves that led to the tumour in his groin. It was a risky procedure because it could cause paralysis below the waist. 'I'm not going anywhere,' said Drew.

The operation took place the next day. It had taken the National Health Service over six months to correctly diagnose Drew's illness but the fact that he was dying finally got him on to the fast track. Everything at their disposal was now devoted to his body's disposal. I went down with him to the theatre. I stood beside his trolley in the busy basement corridor as he scribbled his signature on the consent form. There was a one-in-twenty chance of irreversible haemorrhage. I started to cry when Drew began praying. I ran my hands through his hair. Was this the last time I would see him alive? A gang of builders, in their regulation uniform of jeans, T-shirt, plaid shirt and Caterpillar boots, stopped joshing and stared. Drew disappeared through the swing doors. Our lives had become just another scene from *Casualty*.

Tessa, a nurse who, thus far, had appeared admirably hard-nosed, escorted me back to the ward. Had I thought of counselling? If Drew did not need it, neither did I. The public audience for our private drama was big enough as it was. His parents were sitting by his bed. Jack smiled; Aileen glared.

The operation was successful even though the doctor had to inject the dangerous drugs through the front of Drew: the tumour was so large it blocked the usual approach to the nerves through the back. His team managed to stabilise Drew's blood pressure, bleeding and pain. The morphine dose was halved to 120mg.

*

Leo, from our point of view, was the one ray of sunshine in the dark tunnel of the ward. I had to brace myself each time I entered the Prince Francis: you never knew what you were going to see. When I returned from Burger King, for example, a tall old woman, so thin she could have been a Giacometti figure, stood in the middle of the central aisle, clutching her Zimmer frame, a puddle of shit spreading between her feet. The retired junior-school headmistress did not move. She did not speak. She simply stared straight ahead. I kept walking and, typically British, pretended not to notice. I had my own mess to deal with.

Drew was particularly concerned about the build-up of gas in his stomach. By Thursday morning it was so distended it resembled a basketball. He told Leo he could not pee. The Senior House Officer drew the curtains round his bed and slowly, gently, inserted a catheter. Drew's bladder was empty. I tried to cheer him up: 'My turn now!' Leo said nothing. Drew rolled his eyes.

Although Drew said his right arm made it difficult for him to write, he spent a lot of time scribbling on a pad of Post-It notes. The morphine made him forget things. He wrote down questions that he wished to ask the doctors, the names of all the nurses, the results of his numerous blood tests. He asked me to bring in a film guide and started to compile a list of movies that he wanted to watch again when he went home: *Alien*, *The Thief of Baghdad*, *Bambi*, *An Affair to Remember*, *The African Queen*, *Only Angels Have Wings*, *Arsenic and Old Lace*, *The Man Who Knew Too Much*, the *Back to the Future* trilogy. His favourite film had always been *The Time Machine*. One of his most prized possessions was a signed photo of Rod Taylor. However, there would be no last-reel escape for us.

Drew had an abdominal X-ray after lunch. His condition continued to stabilise. That night, his last in the Middlesex, he had a Badedas bubble-bath. This time we could use the turbo-jets.

Drew had second thoughts about going home right up to the moment of his discharge. He was understandably apprehensive about leaving the hospital, cutting himself off from its resources and staff. Everyone, apart from his parents, persuaded him that it was for the best. The nurses were sweet and supportive. Leo, against all regulations, gave Drew his home number.

So, when the pharmacy delivered his drugs at half-past three, our sorry caravan trailed out of the ward. Drew had amassed a surprising amount of luggage. He held on to his mother's arm as we stood amid the heat and noise of Mortimer Street. A cab soon halted. He went straight to bed when we got in. Aileen did not even take off her coat. She and Jack set off for Camberwell at 5.15. As the silence fell I felt the weight of extra responsibility settle on my shoulders.

We were not alone for long. Cathy, a district nurse, called round to introduce herself. She was closely followed by Drew's GP. There were so many things I wanted to say to him but, for Drew's sake, said nothing.

I unpacked the bags, started on the laundry and tended to Drew's needs. He was snoring when I went to bed. It was heart-breaking to see him lying there, wearing the eye-patch, an anti-thrombosis stocking on his swollen left leg, the morphine pump under his right hand. I left the doors to both our rooms open: the top floor became one large loft space. I slept badly – the open door seemed to invite my nightmare in – but there was no alternative. Drew only woke me once. I gave him a Co-proxamol and some Oramorph, the liquid morphine that Dennis Potter, the playwright, had swigged so spectacularly in his recent, at-death's-door television interview with Melvyn Bragg.

I was vacuuming the hall on Saturday morning when his parents arrived. They were an hour and a half early. It had been weeks since the place had had a good clean: I wanted them to see the flat, Drew's home, at its best. His mother made some sarcastic remark about being house-proud and stepped over the vacuum cleaner. His father followed her upstairs. I carried on cleaning.

The GP called in again. The district nurse changed Drew's pump. Drew threw up twice. He started back on the Cyclizine. I filled the empty shelves in the living room with my film library: videos do tarnish a room.

Jack and Aileen left soon after three. There seemed to me to be no rhyme or reason to their visits, unless they were operating on Australian time. Drew spent ages in the bathroom with the cold tap running. He still had difficulty peeing.

He perked up in the evening and came downstairs. When *The Third Man* had finished he said: 'Here you are.' The tumour on his neck had grown so large that his chain had started to chafe: it was not long enough any more. He unhooked the clasp and placed the crucifix round my neck, sealing it with a kiss. 'You're not going to chicken out, are you?'

'No.' I held the gold cross in my fingers. 'Does this mean you don't believe any more?'

'No. I still believe. I believe He will understand. There's no such place as Hell.'

'There is. This is it.'

'We'll be together again one day. I know it. I'll be waiting for you.' I could feel my eyes begin to prickle. I was sick of crying. It solved nothing.

'Have you decided when?'

'The sooner the better. I'm fed up of waiting. Every day it gets worse and worse. My parents can't take much more. If this goes on they'll have a nervous breakdown.'

'They're not the only ones . . . At least Lumpy can't hurt you any more.'

'No – but his spawn, his evil children, carry on his infernal mission. They're in my liver, my chest, my brain. It's disgusting. Look at me! I've forgotten what it's like to have no pain. We can't let Lumpy win. *I'll* decide when to die, not him.'

'Not tonight though, Possum. I'm not ready.' Now that we were home again I felt stronger, more in control. I wanted us to be together for as long as humanly possible.

'Okay but, remember, you promised. Don't let me down.'

The dog days dragged on. Drew, wearing my old bathrobe, sat on the terrace in the sun. His morphine intake went up and up. It took care of the pains in his back but it also took him further and further into dreamland. His head lolled, his eyes rolled, his lips mouthed silent words. His mother's hostility turned to aggression. The inevitable confrontation finally occurred over Drew's body. We stood on either side of his bed arguing about the best way to look after him.

'I realise you used to be a nurse but in this country the patient's wishes come first. I don't care how you speak to your husband but if you want to remain in this house you'll keep a civil tongue in your head.' Aileen, not surprisingly, hardly spoke to me again. I would have loved to have thrown her out. The Macmillan nurse tried to calm us all down. We had been handed over to the Islington palliative care team now, based at the Royal Free Hospital in Hampstead: the politics, and economics, of pain.

Mandy delivered the 'Octo-pot' we had bought at Camberwell College. I showed it to Drew, made sure he held it in his hands, but it had become a sickening memento of that endless day. Leo and Jenny came round on Tuesday evening. It was strange to see them in casual clothes. The temperature had reached 32 degrees that afternoon: the hottest day of the year so far. After they had spent some time with Drew in his room, we had a bottle of champagne on the terrace. Jack and Aileen stayed upstairs. We discussed the practicalities of ending it all. I asked Leo what would happen if Drew took all his pills.

'He would probably bring them all back up. It's not a good idea.'

That night the heatwave began to break. Blue lightning,

distant thunder, no rain: apocalypse soon. Drew's hiccups plagued him almost as much as his dreams. I stayed with him until each crisis had passed then staggered back to my own bed. We were never more than fifteen feet apart.

He was in the bath when I got up.

'Morning, Possum.' I ran my fingers through his hair. It had not fallen out: in fact it needed cutting. There was no point, though – a horrid thought.

'Did I wake you?'

'Don't think so. D'you want some breakfast?' His torso had shrunk, his stomach was distended and his legs were swollen. It was hard to believe this was the same body that I had so often soaped when we shared a bath. Drew was usually the one in the front: my legs stretched right round him. I like to rest my chin on his shoulder as I hugged him. I crouched down and kissed him on the cheek. It was hollow and bristly. He turned to look at me. The shadows under his eyes had deepened.

'How are you?' He dabbed some bubbles on the end of my nose.

'Okay. And you?'

'The hiccups have stopped for now. I'll try some Shreddies.'

He nearly slipped as he got out of the tub. He was unsteady on his feet and did not come downstairs. The world came to him instead. An endless procession of strange feet trudged up the wooden hill. The district nurse came three times. The Macmillan nurse brought yet another consultant whose compassionate no-nonsense approach was a relief. Even so, it was a shock to hear him discussing Drew's death. Hearing other people talk about it made it seem more real. It also felt like a gross invasion of privacy. So much do-gooding, so little doing good.

His parents and I circled each other uneasily. Jack told me how he had saved Drew's life when he was two years old. He had given his baby son the kiss of life when he stopped breathing in his cot. The closed curtains in Drew's room made the sunshine behind them seem even brighter. It was hot beneath the roof. The two old Pifco fans that I had found in the sale-rooms at the top of the road whirred away furiously. The telephone remained silent.

At half-past six the doorbell rang. It was Elaine, on her way home from *Time Out*. She dumped two carrier-bags of food from M&S in the hall and put her arms around me. Such a sign of affection produced the now automatic response.

'I'm sorry. I can't help it. I know crying makes me look even worse.'

'Impossible.'

'I can't go on like this. I can't.' I did not want to let go of her. I let go.

'How is he?'

'They said he's unlikely to see next week. But they said that last week too.'

'And his parents?'

'At this rate they'll be lucky to see next week as well. His mother slipped on the stairs this afternoon. Serves her right for wearing pop-sox.'

As I put the ready meals in the fridge I realised they had a longer use-by date than Drew.

I closed the door behind his parents and rested my forehead against the warm wood. I am not sure how long I stayed like that. The next thing I knew the phone was ringing and Drew was yelling for me to answer it. Marta was calling to say that she and Pascal were moving from Paris to London for good. I tried to sound delighted.

I heated up some tagliatelle and ate it sitting on the stairs so I could watch TV and keep an eye on Drew at the same time. He seemed to have gone back to sleep. When I had cleared up I lay on the sofa in his room and watched the light slowly fade. At the back of the house, kids played soccer until they could no longer see the ball. At the front, cabs revved and braked, revved and braked as they negotiated the speed bumps, jolting awake the sozzled bankers inside.

Drew's breathing became more and more erratic. Just when it seemed that he had stopped breathing, his lungs would wheeze into action. It was known as the Cheyne–Stokes syndrome. It was impossible not to listen to it.

Drew sat up. 'Horrible! Horrible!' My blood ran cold. I rushed to his side.

'What is it? What's the matter?' I hoped it was just a bad dream.

'Why am I like this, Mark? I hurt. I hurt.'

'Where's the pain?'

'My head, my heart, my back.' He began to cry. I held him

so long I thought he had gone to sleep. He had not. 'Oh make it stop, make it stop.'

'D'you want a booster?'

'I'll do it.' He pressed the pump. He lay down again. 'Don't leave me.'

'I won't. You know I won't. Not ever.' I held his hand. No one should have to suffer this much. I had postponed the inevitable for too long. My selfishness sickened me. It was time to keep my promise.

The clock of St Mary's struck three. Over two hours had passed in what felt like seconds. Drew was still awake.

'D'you want a Temazepam?'

'Please.' I fetched him one of mine: they were stronger than his. I was not sure I could go through with it if he were awake. He closed his eyes. I stroked his arm. The half-hour chimed. My heart began to thud.

I let go of his hand and stood up slowly. 'Drew?' There was no reply to my whisper. I crept into my bedroom and picked up the pillow. It somehow did not seem right to use one of his. I was afraid the thumping in my chest would wake him. This was not me. It was someone else in a parallel universe. They were about to do something I would never do. The air on the top floor became hotter and heavier. I held my breath.

The scenario I envisaged harked back to the climax of *Betty Blue* in which a novelist suffocates his lover after she has gone mad and blinded herself. However, I had overlooked one crucial fact: Betty was strapped to her bed.

I kissed Drew goodbye. Then, gripping the pillow in both hands, I placed it over his face and pressed down firmly.

'I love you, Drew. I will always love you.' His hands shot up and grabbed my wrists. His strength was astonishing. I whipped the pillow away. His blue eyes bored into mine. Shock and terror were mixed with sheer rage.

At that moment I experienced true horror for the first time. Nothing that had gone before had prepared me for it. I felt something give inside, a sort of dull crack and an icy blackness bloomed in my brain. Vertigo, panic, desire and relief welled up. I burst into tears.

'I thought that that was what you wanted.' I flung my arms round his neck and sobbed my heart out. Now he would think I wished him dead.

'Not yet. Not yet. I'll let you know when, somehow.' I could not stop shaking. Was I going mad? The notion suddenly seemed attractive. There appeared to be no other means of escape – except that I could not leave Drew behind. He held me as I wept. 'There, there, my poor baby.'

All this time I had been under the impression that I was looking after him but, in reality, it was the other way round. He, as usual, was looking after me.

I did not sleep. I stayed beside Drew and watched over him. I was there when incontinence finally arrived. The pads that had been provided were pretty useless so I switched to the condom that led, via a tube, to a bag. It had to be kept in place with adhesive tape.

The district nurse added a sedative to the morphine in the pump. Drew gave up eating solids. His mother made him junket, which he had loved as a child. It was little different from the Ensure that the hospital had given us: insipid liquid meals in tiny cartons. Survival rations.

Drew continued to fight the cancer. It was as if he still hoped for a last-minute miracle. He seemed to fade in front of my eyes. He was ineffably brave. On Friday he stopped taking anything by mouth. We used miniature sponges on plastic sticks to moisten his lips. I kept on talking to him but did not expect him to answer. I jumped when he suddenly stroked my cheek and said: 'Hello.'

'Hello.' I tried to smile.

'Now. Do it now.'

'I can't. Your parents are still here. As soon as they've gone.'

It was our last day together. The fact that time stood still was no consolation: Drew was waiting to die. I swung between panic and determination every few minutes. I had to go through with it. It would be the ultimate proof of how much I loved him.

The planet spun on. The 'cash for questions' scandal raged in Westminster; Tony Blair appeared to be leading John Prescott in the race for leadership of the Labour Party; Brazil and Italy would meet in the World Cup Final in Pasadena on Sunday. It was all utterly irrelevant. Only Drew mattered.

I drifted round the flat. Police horses from the local stables clopped past. I could not hear the sound without thinking of the coconut shells we had played with at infant school: 'Horsey, Horsey, don't you stop/Just let your feet go clippety-clop.' Even then I had wondered if I would fall in love and get married like Mummy and Daddy. Well, it had taken a quarter of a century but I had found my true love. Now I had to kill him.

I relived our first meeting at the Barbican, the trip to Nice and the cruise. I chatted to Drew about our visit to Stratford, the wet weekend on the Grand Union Canal and my birthday at Amberley Castle. We had managed to do a lot in a short time yet I still felt we had been cheated. Drew squeezed my hand. Aileen was in the doorway. I let her take my place.

The Macmillan nurse asked me if I needed a night-sitter. 'You look as if you could do with some sleep.'

'I'll sleep when it's over.' We had seen too many strangers in the past week.

'It shouldn't be much longer. He's put up such a fight.' She picked up her bag. 'I like coming here. This house is full of love. Drew's very lucky to have you.'

I was terrified his parents would insist on staying the night. In the end they left just before half-past ten. Aileen, as usual, told Drew to 'take care of you for me'. They seemed so vulnerable as they walked up Packington Street, his father still wearing his Akubra hat and shorts with knee-length socks. They would attract some looks on the bus back to Camberwell.

I locked the door. There was no way out. I had to keep my promise. Half of me had been secretly hoping that it would be too late. On the other hand, the thought of Drew dying in the belief that I had failed him at the vital moment was unbearable. I climbed the stairs. It did not seem a second since we had followed the estate agent up the same steps.

I fetched my pillow. I watched myself as, way down below, I walked into his bedroom. I lit the scented candle that had flickered through each night. Five minutes more: I would just sit with him for five more minutes. I held his hand. I could not believe it when St Mary's struck midnight. Time had telescoped.

'Drew? Can you hear me?' He moved his lips but no sound came out. 'Blink once for yes.' He blinked.

'Do you still want me to keep my promise?'

Blink.

'I'm going to ask you twelve times. Blink twice if you change your mind. Do you want me to help you die right now?'

Blink.

After the third time I just said, 'Right now?' Each time Drew blinked. After the tenth time I paused. If he blinked in the next few seconds I would not go through with it. He might have been dreaming or subconsciously maintaining a rhythm. He did not blink.

'Right now?'

Blink.

'Right now?'

Blink.

I waited for another blink. I prayed for another blink. Drew simply gazed into my eyes. If I waited any longer it would be torture for the both of us. I kissed him. His breath smelled of death.

'Hold on to my wrists. I love you, Drew.'

It was easier the second time. We both knew what to

expect. I pressed down so hard I was afraid I would break his nose. He was much weaker now but the strength of his resistance still surprised me. It was pure reflex. It had to be: his instinct for survival overrode his will. I kept the pillow there long after the bucking had stopped.

When I eventually removed it, and flung it to the floor, his mouth was open. I closed it and kissed him goodnight. I undressed and lay on my stomach beside him, my right arm across his chest. It was over. At last it was over. I felt nothing at all. My other self, high above, watched over us. I fell asleep.

10

AFTERWARDS

Your life can end at any moment, whether you want it to or not. Drew did not take the easy way out. He waited till death was imminent and inevitable. Cancer was killing him, the morphine was killing him, but he denied victory to them both. His last hours were defiant proof of our enduring love. Love cannot conquer everything. It can, however, endure.

I woke from a deep, dreamless sleep at around half-past four. It was unnaturally quiet. Drew's eyes were open.

'Drew? Drew? Drew!' I put my ear to his chest. It was cold. Nothing. I felt for a pulse. Nothing. I was in bed with a corpse. I lifted the towel that lay across his groin. Constipation was no longer a problem. The district nurse had warned me what would happen. I put my arms round Drew and cried — but not very much. The tears, for once, would not come. 'What am I going to do without you?' I was in shock. Was Drew really dead? I checked again. He was so cold.

I took refuge in action. There was a mess to clear up. The pads had done their work. I talked to Drew as I sponged him clean. His bottom was virtually the only part of his body that had not changed. It was still smooth, firm and chunky. 'It's yours, all yours,' he had whispered in Nice. I would never touch it again. I kissed him goodbye on both cheeks.

The grief came in waves. Each time it hit me I would cry for a few seconds then stop. Drew's eyes would not stay closed. He was proud of their blueness but his offer to donate them had been refused. I placed silver coins on their lids. I made some coffee and waited till half-past five to call his parents. They arrived within the hour. Aileen put her arms round me in the hall. All three of us wept. I let them go upstairs alone. The shrieks that followed made the hairs on the back of my neck stand up.

At 7.30 I bleeped Drew's GP. I helped Aileen put a pair of boxer shorts on her son. He was already stiff. The fact that the shorts were mine, a Christmas present from my grandmother, was somehow pleasing. The doctor, before he came through the door, crushed a dog-end on the step. He wore socks with his sandals. He hauled himself up to Drew's room for the last time. I watched as he fished a stethoscope out of his black bag and listened to Drew's chest in three places. He gazed into Drew's eyes with an ophthalmoscope. I went downstairs to call the undertaker.

Two men, their faces composed into masks of professional

solemnity, hefted Drew into a reusable coffin. The smallest room of all. They replaced the lid, fitted a black nylon pall over the brown fibreglass box, and tipped Drew upright. The stairs creaked as the three of them made their way down. When they reached the hall the men returned Drew to the horizontal. I opened the front door. As the coffin passed I tapped on the lid and said, 'Bye, Possum.' He was slid into the back of the black Volkswagen van and, at five past ten, was driven away for ever.

His parents left twenty minutes later. I was alone. I went back to Drew's room. When I snuffed the candle I blew too hard and spattered the curtains and carpet with wax. The stains remain to this day.

I was surprised that the world was still there when I opened the curtains: the viewer, not the view, had changed. Once I would have said the events of that morning had seemed unreal. However, there is nothing more real than death. The scales had fallen from my eyes. I was seeing the world as it truly was for the very first time. I had thought it one kind of place when, in fact, it was quite another.

Henceforth love, success and happiness were what other people enjoyed. I had been lucky enough to have shared all three with Drew but they, too, had gone out of the door for good – or so I thought. I had to remember that some people never got to experience them. It did not make me feel any better though. My only consolation was that the worst possible thing that could have happened had happened. It was this that gave me the strength to carry on.

I stripped the bed. Drew was dead. I knew it but did not

feel it. The numbness made it easier for me to make the unavoidable telephone calls. If it is hard to receive such terrible news it is equally hard to accept the automatic expressions of sympathy. I did not want other people's pity: I wanted Drew back. I thought of him lying in a fridge at the undertaker's. He was literally round the corner in Essex Road. Naked and surrounded by strangers. I ought to be with him. 'You are,' said my other self. 'He never left you. His body may have gone but Drew is still with you. He's here in this room. He's in your head and in your heart.'

I was beside myself. I still could not quite believe that I had done what I had done. Someone else had suffocated Drew. Someone braver and stronger: a romantic hero, not a neurotic wreck. Someone who could risk their own neck for the sake of a dying lover. It was not so much a question of being caught as being able to live with the consequences. His only reward was the knowledge that, at the most, he had spared Drew twelve or twenty-four more hours of anguish. No one can feel another's pain. Each time I tried to imagine what Drew must have been going through, my mind went blank. Waiting to die as your body disintegrated about you: that defined 'degrading'.

The district nurse came round to collect the left-over apparatus of palliative care. I helped her load the fleecy underblanket (to prevent bedsores), the metal cage (to keep sheets off the feet), the yellow mini swing-bin for used hypodermics and all the boxes and bottles of drugs – but not the Sevredol and Diazepam – into her car. The happy pills were bound to come in useful later.

I had a long, hot bath and tried to unclench. Every part of me ached: stomach, head, heart, arms, legs. I slept in my own bed for a couple of hours. There was no milk. I walked up the road to buy some, unable to meet anyone's eye. Could they tell what had happened just by looking at me?

When darkness eventually fell I toasted Drew's memory. The champagne had lost its taste. I watched 'Masonic Mysteries', my favourite episode of *Inspector Morse*. I was afraid to go to bed. I was alone: the consultants, doctors, nurses, auxiliaries and porters were dealing with the next in line. No one needed me to fetch something, hold something or sign something. The waiting was over. Drew's room was empty. What was I going to do now?

I put a photograph of Drew in the frame that I had bought him for Christmas and placed it beside my bed. It was the one I had taken on the cruise. Two snips removed the girls from the picture. I blew him a kiss and turned out the light. Grief swept over me as soon as my head touched the pillow. The darkness swirled in my mind. Drew was dead. I might as well be too. I could sense myself becoming unhinged. I had struggled to keep myself together for Drew's sake. I had no reason to any more. I had no reason at all.

The phrase 'mad with grief' conjures up images of screaming mouths, flailing fists, tearing hair and gnashing teeth, but I lost my mind slowly and quietly. The fact that I had helped Drew die did not worry me. I was proud that, in the end, I had been able to keep my promise. Drew was dead. I was not. Somehow I had to go on living without him. The past three months had been an eternity of pain and waiting that had nevertheless flown by. The cancer had brought chaos to our lives. What I needed now was order and stability.

On Monday morning I collected Drew's death certificate from the doctors' surgery. When I said Drew's name the women behind the counter in Reception stopped gossiping and turned round. One of them handed me the form. 'We're very sorry.'

'Thank you. So am I.'

I walked down to Finsbury Town Hall in Rosebery Avenue. I never expected to enter the Register Office – Drew and I would not have been allowed to stand on its steps in a blizzard of confetti – yet here I was in the wood-panelled room watching as our names were linked for ever. Mr Koch used a fountain pen to record the details of Drew's demise in the big black book. Black ink did not fade. They had used biros in the 1970s: the pages were virtually blank today. A whole generation had paled into nothingness. Drew's GP had misspelled 'melanoma' but it was illegal to change a single letter of the cause of death: the error had to stand.

I was given a green form that allowed the undertaker to proceed with the cremation. The thought of the cancer being consumed by fire was deeply satisfying. I wandered back to Essex Road in the sunshine, surprised to see my own shadow. I felt hollow, absent. The office at the funeral parlour had wainscoting too. It was merely a larger version of the wooden boxes in the workshop at the rear. I tried not to think of Drew laid out a couple of rooms away.

The undertaker had been shocked when, the previous week, I had asked how much the cheapest possible funeral was: 'No one's ever asked me that before!' I explained that Drew's parents wanted to take the ashes back to Australia. None of us wished to prolong the agony by having a church ceremony here – they planned instead to have a memorial service in Cairns.

That night I dreamed about Drew. We were hugging and crying: something was wrong. I woke up in a panic. His parents were due at 9.30. I had half an hour to go through Drew's things. They were bound to be early.

Apart from the bed, I had left everything as it was. The room was a minefield of memories. However, unless I acted now, I would have little to remember him by except his crucifix. I felt like a burglar. I managed to grab his home videos, his favourite Sportscraft sweater – 'Made in Australia' – the HOT and COLD cufflinks and his wallet before the doorbell rang.

Jack and Aileen shed a few tears before setting to work. The tension and anger between us had vanished. We were three strangers united by our love for one man. No one expects to outlive their children. The Morgans were going through a harrowing time. If they wished to blame me for what had happened I no longer cared: their resentment could not affect my ability to look after Drew now. Besides, in some ways they would be right to do so. It was because of me that Drew was in England, at the mercy of the NHS, and I, along with the chemotherapy and morphine, had hastened his death. None of us, their son included, could have gone on much longer. Drew was aware of this and, selfless to the end, put us all out of our misery. He allowed me one final demonstration of my love. His life had an active conclusion, not a passive petering-out. Sometimes the wrong move is the right one.

His parents packed as much as they could into Drew's empty cases. Qantas, in such circumstances, granted the bereaved an extra weight allowance. Debbie and Simon both worked for the airline. Aileen sorted through Drew's clothes and offered me the occasional item. Adrian, his nephew, would be able to wear most of them until he shot up again. Jack sat at the computer and tried to explain some of its more advanced functions. He had two of his own at home. Fortunately, he had no need of another and, anyway, it was too big to carry. I suggested he take the zip-drive and all the software: I would never use them.

They managed to fit three-quarters of Drew's belongings into his suitcases, briefcase and rucksack. The whole process seemed distasteful and premature. It was too early to be picking over the remains. However, the Morgans simply wanted to return to Australia as soon as possible – and take as much of their son with them as they could. My old bathrobe and a packet of cotton-buds disappeared along with Drew's watch, camera and camcorder. It was only much later that I realised the video of Amberley Castle must have still been in the machine. Drew was the ghost now.

I helped Jack put the luggage in a cab and waved them off. It was after one o'clock but they had not even had a drink. I was unwashed, unshaven and shaking. A kindly neighbour offered me her condolences in grotesque officialese. It was the first time we had spoken. Elsie, from downstairs, had played hell with me the day before: 'Why didn't you tell us? Arthur was very upset.' I did not want to talk about it.

Drew was cremated on Wednesday 20 July, my father's fifty-eighth birthday. Cards and letters continued to arrive, including one from my parents, signed, as always, by my mother. I had hoped she would come down to London but, when I invited her to stay, she said she could not leave my father. I was not going to beg. Jane, the Macmillan nurse, wrote in a schoolgirl script: 'You cared for Drew so well, he died with peace and dignity. You showed great love and respect for him.' Was that true? A friend of Drew's in Brisbane sent a basket of yellow chrysanthemums. Fiona, his boss, sent me a copy of the obituary she had written for 'Axis', the weekly office newsletter:

It is with great sadness that I write to tell you of the death of Drew Morgan. Drew lost his battle with cancer three months after it was first diagnosed. During that time he went through a lot of pain and disappointment as one set of treatment after another failed to bring about any improvement in his condition, in fact some treatments made his day-to-day condition much worse. Throughout he displayed exceptional courage and good humour, always showing more concern for family and friends than for himself. When I last saw him he had less than one to month to live, yet he still asked about all his friends at work and insisted on making arrangements to come and say 'goodbye'. Unfortunately, he never made it – he died in his sleep, at home in London, just one week after leaving hospital. Drew was only with the Project for fifteen months but, in that time, people came to depend on him, not just for the excellent work he did, but also as a friend. We are sure his gentle, easy-going ways, matched with his professionalism, will be missed by all those who knew him.

Several well-wishers assured me that 'life must go on'. I was not so sure. Every day I had to force myself to get up and get out of the house. The simplest tasks took hours. I had my hair cut off. Richard was the only heterosexual male stylist I had encountered: I called him Straight Dick. He agreed the crew-cut suited me. It symbolised my grave new world – and disguised the first few grey hairs.

At 4pm the next day – three months exactly since Drew was told he had two years to live – I collected him from the undertaker's. A box full of dust. The address was wrong on the certificate of cremation: we did not live in Packington Square. It did not even prove to be the last entry in an epic catalogue of errors. I ordered a single red rose to be sent to the Morgans' address in Cairns on 12 August, the day of his memorial service. Even though I made the order four days in advance Drew's brother later told me that the flower had been delivered on the thirteenth. Perhaps I was old-fashioned in expecting people to get things right.

Drew felt like a child-in-arms as I carried him down the road. I weighed the plastic bronze urn on the electronic scales we had bought in Selfridges: 6lbs 2¾oz, or 2.8kg. I braced myself and lifted the lid. Grey flakes, white powder: an obscene porridge.

His parents were due at five. I carried Drew round the flat so that he could say goodbye to each room – we had made love in all of them. I felt angry rather than foolish. I was not talking to myself. I sat on the terrace until the door-bell rang. A sparrowhawk alighted on a chimney-pot on top of the council flats. I had not seen one round here before. Drew would have been able to tell me what the bird signified in Roman mythology. A parting soul? No, just a feathered lizard on the look-out for prey.

Jack was on time and alone. He stayed less than five minutes. The boy who once drank only Mateus Rosé went off with his father in a Bibendum carrier-bag. It was a good name for a vintner. Aileen made a farewell call from Heathrow on Sunday morning. It ended with both of us in tears.

I drank a lot during the following weeks. Friends came round with bottles and cheques: they kept a glass in my hand and a roof over my head. Alcohol released my demons. Each would-be comforter sat on a sofa and listened as I talked and cried till the small hours. However, if I tried to tell them what had really happened, they suddenly became restless and deaf. The truth can be a dangerous thing. I decided to bury it.

Howard was due to start at Hurstpierpoint College in September. I helped the new Head of Classics move his and Sarah's belongings from West Hampstead to West Sussex. It was an opportunity to leave London behind, a summer holiday by stealth. The route we took in the hired Luton van to Burgess Hill was virtually the same as the one we had taken on our way to Amberley. The three of us went swimming at Climping, admired the length of the Long Man at Wilmington but spent most of our time eating and drinking: lunch on Worthing Pier, afternoon tea at Ockenden Manor, cocktails at the Grand Hotel in Brighton, dinner at Little Thakeham – a country house designed by Lutyens – and, if we did not go out, champagne barbecues in the back garden. The hangovers could not make me feel any worse than I already did. I was jealous of Howard and Sarah's coupledom yet admired their willingness to move on. I knew, had always known, that I would not move out of Packington Street. We had been at our happiest and unhappiest there. I was not going to let anyone else sleep in Drew's room. If I had to leave, it would be in the same manner as Drew.

I tried to sweat off the effects of the alcohol at the gym. I did not want to go, but it was a good way of establishing a daily routine. There were times, as I walked past the doctors' surgery to the Tube, that I felt like sinking to the ground and staying there. I stopped in my tracks on a few

occasions but something – anger? embarrassment? curiosity? – always made me carry on. The receptionist, when she
handed over my new membership card in return for Drew's
old one, told me that another Mark Sanderson belonged to
the gym. He lived in Kentish Town. I hoped he was having a
better life.

Thus far I had only used the pool there – if I wanted to use
the gym equipment I would have to undergo a fitness assess-
ment. My instructor was a South African boy called Bill. He
had melting brown eyes but I did not feel even a flicker of
lust. Bill inhabited a different world. His friendly youthfulness
emphasised the gulf between us. At thirty-two I felt old,
worn out, ready for the knacker's yard. Middle age had
arrived early. I even started to read the death notices in *The
Times*.

At the end of August I returned to Wraysbury, the scene of
the bonfire party in 1992. I had written to the Clerk of
Justices at High Wycombe explaining that Drew would be
unable to pay the speeding fine because he was dead. The
house was about to be demolished: a cul-de-sac of 'executive
homes' would be built over its kitchen garden, rose garden,
croquet lawn and orchard. Charles's father had killed himself
in the master bedroom – whisky, barbiturates, a plastic bag –
and his son was marking the impending, if lucrative, destruc-
tion of his childhood home with a series of parties. At
midnight a group of us went skinny-dipping in the nearby
lake. It was actually a flooded gravel pit, but it made no

difference. There was a full moon; the heat of the day still lingered; and the jets from Heathrow had finally stopped screaming overhead. I was too drunk and dizzy with Diazepam to care whether or not I drowned. In fact I hoped I would.

The cold, silky water made my hot skin shrink. It was exhilarating. We appeared to be swimming through quicksilver. One of the guests raced me to the island. He was called Philippe. We stood on the shore panting, shivering and laughing. We had sex. For the first time in weeks, I felt alive. There was no guilt the next day. I had not been unfaithful to Drew. I had not defiled his memory. He would have approved.

Philippe reminded me that I had not just lost Drew, I had also lost the intimacy between us. Drew was so much in my thoughts that I had hardly begun to miss him physically. Every so often I would find myself thinking, 'Oh, I must tell Drew that,' only for the sickening truth to sink in once again. It was as if my mind refused to accept it. I did everything possible to minimise his absence. I wore one of his shirts even though it was too small, I used his Armani aftershave, I even left *Neighbours* on in the background because it was a comfort to hear an Australian accent. I spent a whole afternoon playing and replaying the tape on the answering machine in a futile attempt to hear Drew's voice. All his messages had been erased.

I should never have asked Mandy to move in with me. It went against all my instincts but I was desperate. I could not continue to rely on hand-outs from my friends and I could not find a job. *Woman's Own*, the Channel 4 press office and even the public relations department at Lloyds Bank turned me down: I had too many qualifications and too little experience. I was too old and therefore too expensive. If I was not going to move out of Packington Street then someone had to move in.

She stayed for five days. Mandy was a loyal and loving friend but I could not live with her. We were totally out of sync. On the second evening I waited hours to have dinner with her as planned only for her to turn up having already eaten. On the fourth evening I came home to find wine trickling out of a frozen bottle in the freezer compartment and a strange man's jacket on the banister. She was perfectly entitled to have overnight guests – it was, after all, now her home as well – but it was far too soon for me to share my space, to relinquish control over my surroundings. I had not recovered from the last wave of invasions. I developed a bunker mentality. The flat was my refuge. My suspicions were right: if I could not be alone in it with Drew I would go mad. The débâcle proved that the threat of a nervous breakdown had by no means receded.

It was an ignoble way to repay Mandy's generosity and support. I felt doubly guilty because she had been glad to quit her flat in Camberwell. Now she had to find somewhere else to live.

Mandy's imminent arrival had forced me to clear out Drew's room. I had not touched the things left behind by his parents.

Now I had another mess to sort out. I knew it would hurt. I found some strange metal loops called 'Wonder Buttons'. They claimed to 'l-o-o-s-e-n tight collars'. The tumour on his neck must have caused more trouble than he had admitted. I took the few remaining clothes to Oxfam and Fiona took the books on 'Historic Swindon' back to Reading: 'They'll make his colleagues laugh.' She told me how Drew's trousers had once split at work. Staples had closed the gaping seam. The onlookers had enjoyed his mortification most of all. A couple of weeks later he had joined the gym and started taking health supplement pills. I could not bear to throw out the brown jars of spirulina and kava kava root.

The bedside cabinet held a treasure trove. Captain Morgan had hoarded everything – and kept quiet about it. He was forever complaining about my mania for tidying up and throwing things away. Postcards, love letters, birthday cards; theatre programmes, menus, tickets; souvenir bookmarks, hotel bills and hospital appointments. The residue of our whole relationship was here from the Mayan death mask in the Hayward Gallery to the Ashton Memorial in Lancaster. I did not realise it at the time, but he had bequeathed this book to me.

There were a couple of other surprises. Drew had kept in touch with Nathan, the psychiatrist he had met in Hawaii. In one of the letters, Nathan invited Drew and I to stay with him and his boyfriend in Euclid. What had they got up to in Honolulu? I hoped they had enjoyed themselves. The possibility that Drew might have been unfaithful did not bother me. His life was so short that I hoped he had made the most of every opportunity. It was more likely that Drew, in spite of his libido, had remained true to himself and me. I considered writing to his American friend but eventually discarded the idea.

The second surprise was a genuine shock. At a quiet moment during one of his all-night shifts, Drew, like many bored office workers, must have had some fun with the black-and-white photocopier. He had Xeroxed his face and hands. A palmist could have told his fortune from the result. Each line on his hand, each bristle on his chin, each pore on his nose was clearly visible. His nails had not been bitten then. According to the watch on his left wrist it had been 5.16 on a Wednesday morning. What had happened to the leather bracelet on his wrist? He had not worn it in hospital. The flash had given his flesh a horrid white pallor. The picture of him open-mouthed made me gasp. His lips formed a gaping black hole. It looked like a death mask. I burst into tears. I put my palms on top of his. The paper was cold too.

Sally Payne saved my skin. When the TV Editor of the *Sunday Times* asked me to preview some programmes once again I told her about my plight. She offered me work as a freelance sub-editor. It was boring but well-paid: £17.80 an hour. I could not afford to say no.

In those days the newspaper was housed in a long, low warehouse just inside the compound of Fortress Wapping. Little more than a tunnel, it had been built, fittingly enough, by prisoners of the Napoleonic Wars. A stint on the dreaded treadmill could not have been as exhausting as an eight-hour shift hunched over a clapped-out keyboard. The work was unchallenging but required total concentration. I was familiar with the Atex computer system because I had used it at *Time Out*. The television schedules came down the line from Broadcasting Data Services. Our task was to convert them into the newspaper's house style and ensure each file was the correct length to fill its allotted space on the page. This involved turning the programme billings into recognisable English – for example, 'Sharon falls out with Phil' – high-lighting films by putting them in boxes, adding cross-references to Critics' Choices – the previews on the opposite page – working out Videoplus numbers if they were missing, and putting the various symbols for Stereo, Subtitles and Repeats in the correct order. Widows, lone words on a line of their own, had to be avoided at all times. I, too, tried not to stand out.

The TV section operated from Sunday to Wednesday; news subs used the desks from Thursday to Saturday. The second half of our week was mainly spent adding late changes to the schedules and proofing the TV, radio and satellite pages for all nine editions of the newspaper. The television guide in the 'Culture' section of the *Sunday Times* had to be the best and most accurate free guide available.

After a fortnight my left shoulder hurt so much that I thought I would have to quit. It felt as though someone were twisting a knife into it. Stretching had little effect on the repetitive strain but popping a Nurofen every three hours dulled the pain. The work was exquisite punishment for a presumptuous writer. The cramped subbing station afforded me views of the whole news department. The excitable journalists played like kids in a sand-pit. The senior editors returned from extended lunches with flushed cheeks and armfuls of freebies. The deputy editor seemed to receive extravagant bouquets every day. We hardly ever took breaks and made do with what was on the trolley that came round each weekday morning and afternoon: pre-packed sandwiches, salads, crisps, canned drinks and chocolate bars. When the scrawny middle-aged woman rang her bicycle-bell and squawked 'Trolley! Trolley!' hacks would scurry down the aisles from all sides and descend on her like a flock of seagulls. The muffins on sale were the same brand as those sold in the Middlesex Hospital.

I went to the gym each morning then walked past the Tower of London and through St Katharine's Dock to Wapping. The routine lent my life a structure. I appeared to be holding down a job, and holding myself together, but it did not feel like that inside. My heart sank as I walked back to the empty flat. The lights were on timer-switches. As I came along Raleigh Street I could see the lamp in Drew's room shining in the dark. The leak had returned with the first of the autumn storms. The stain on his ceiling got bigger.

I often dreamed about Drew. We would be hugging and crying and I would tell him that I would do anything to bring him back. I slept badly, frequently lying awake between 4 and 5am. I wondered if this was the hour in which Drew would have died: it was when the human spirit was supposed to be at its lowest. Elaine said it was a sign of depression. Of course I was depressed: I was bereaved. It was only natural.

I felt both too much and too little. It was as if I were hypersensitive and dead at the same time. The Heddonists took me to the Chelsea Arts Club on my birthday. They had something else to celebrate too: Panoptic had been commissioned to turn another of my programme ideas into a six-part series. 'Out of Order' featured two opponents apparently stuck in a lift for fifteen minutes. My four-figure fee was a godsend but, as the champagne cocktails took effect, I realised there could be no end to my nightmare. Until that moment it seemed that I had been getting somewhere: each day that passed brought me closer to a resolution. However, I was longing for an impossible reunion. Drew was not in hospital or in Australia. There was no point crossing off the days because he was never coming home. I put my head on the table and cried and cried. I could not stop. I was as close to hysteria as I had ever been. I could not have cared less that I was making a scene. Michael and Mary took me home.

Three days later, on 19 November, Alex celebrated his birthday with dinner for twenty in a Kensington restaurant. I had to force myself to go. 'You'll enjoy it,' said Alex. 'There'll be lots of available men.'

It was the ordeal I had anticipated. Steven, after offering his commiserations, seemed to want to form a joyless widows' club. While we had both lost our partners, mutual support groups were not my kind of thing. The other guests kept saying that I simply must see *Four Weddings and a Funeral*. I was in no mood for a romantic comedy although I had already looked up the Auden poem that everyone was so fond of quoting. 'Funeral Blues' may not have been his greatest work but it epitomised how I felt:

He was my North, my South, my East and West,
My working week, and my Sunday rest,
My noon, my midnight, my talk, my song;
I thought love would last for ever: I was wrong.

I wished I had written it.

The first ever National Lottery Draw took place that evening. I based my six numbers on the dates of Drew's birthday and my own (reversing the years). It was about time I had some good luck. Blind Fortune did not think so. My grandmother thought that she might win because 19 November was her birthday as well. I told her we Scorpios should know better than to believe in astrology. Her response was uncharacteristically sardonic: 'It has as much meaning as anything else.'

I had last seen her in October. I took her a bunch of copper chrysanthemums. When she went into the kitchen to put them in water I examined the collection of drugs that had joined the bowl of fruit and wedding photograph on the sideboard. Some of the names were sickeningly familiar: Co-danthramer, Dexamethasone, Sevredol. My grandmother, however, looked much the same as she had at Christmas. I admired the fact that she was still managing on her own in the house that she had lived in for more than half a century.

The next time I saw Em was Friday 23 December. I did not recognise her. I had finished at the *Sunday Times* on the Wednesday and caught the train up to Lancaster with Howard the following day. My grandmother was now in St John's. The hospice was in a peaceful, wooded location down by the canal. I reached her bedside just after 11am. Her breathing was very poor. Presently she opened her eyes and held out her hand. It was cold and clammy. She insisted on putting her teeth in. I opened her Christmas card for her. Our eyes met. I kissed her goodbye. She died ten minutes later.

My mother was an only child — perhaps this is what has made her tough. She comforted my sister and me more than we could comfort her. She appeared not to need to talk about what was most important. I had tried and failed to talk to her about Drew, about being gay, on the telephone: I could sense her becoming tight-lipped. It was determination rather than denial. Chatter never changed anything.

I went with my mother to register the death. While we waited for the office in Queen Square to re-open after lunch we browsed in a second-hand bookshop round the corner. I found a first edition of *My Secret History* by Paul Theroux, complete with dust-jacket, priced at £2. My mother gave me the money: 'It's Christmas.' The Registrar's words were virtually identical to those used by Mr Koch in July. Each death was unique but the bureaucracy remained the same.

The festive season delayed the obsequies. I seemed to have spent the whole year waiting in dread. One morning my father told me I had been shouting in my sleep: 'I couldn't make out what you were saying. It sounded like "You! You! You!"' He was wrong. It was not the first time I had woken up crying, 'Drew!'

A week later my grandmother's funeral service was held in the ancient Priory where she had married my grandfather, Linda had married Craig and I had sung in the school choir. I would not have got through it without Drew's Diazepam. The guilt continued to mount up: her death was not affecting me as much as it should because I was still numb. I should have visited my grandmother more often. I should not have blurted out the truth: instead of helping my mother I had increased her burden. She came with me to the station after the wake. It was the first time she had ever seen me off. Perhaps she was trying to tell me something.

There was a Christmas card from Drew's parents among the pile of mail. I had sent cards to all his family: I was not going to let them forget me. I had to convince them that Drew and I were not merely having a fling. The scene on the card showed sunrise over the peaks of Mount Barney in southern Queensland. His mother had written the message:

Dear Mark, we hope your life is back on track, and the sadness of 1994 behind you. I imagine you will be spending the holiday season with your family, a time to recharge your batteries and look forward. Take care Mark. Best wishes, Aileen and Jack.

Back on track? If only. I was glad that 1994 was almost over. It had been a true *annus horribilis*. However, the next three years would not be much better. My life was about to go off the rails completely.

II

DOWNWARDS

Personal happiness is said to depend on three things: lover, home, job. I had lost the first and would lose the second if I quit the third. At the end of January I left the *Sunday Times*. It was not the pain in my shoulder, the frequent migraines or the boredom: it was grief. I had tried to carry on, to pick up the pieces, to pretend that I was on the up – but I was not. The strain of the past six months had drained me. I had nothing left to draw upon. I wanted to die.

The knot of cold dread in my stomach never went away. I was constantly tired. Dreams tormented me each night. In one I was asked if I wished to hold the urn at Drew's memorial service: 'Please. It's so long since I held him in my arms.' In another I was in the arms of a handsome doctor but tore myself away: Drew was waiting for me outside the room; Drew was cross with me, he would not hug me, and when, finally, he did, I woke up. I had not died of heartbreak: did this mean I did not love him enough?

I stopped going to the gym. What was the point? It was too late to leave a beautiful corpse. I itched and shook all the time. My friends split into two camps. The women gathered round; the men left me to stew. 'I don't know what to do,' said Alex, full of his new French boyfriend. 'You're wallowing in grief.' I was not wallowing: I was drowning.

The fact that I *knew* I was going out of my mind only made matters worse. On the other hand, I was afraid of waking up one morning completely mad and knowing nothing about it. I had to do something. I made an appointment to see my GP. The ostensible reason for my visit was to get some more eczema cream but, even though she was being shadowed by a medical student, I burst into tears. I explained how I felt. I could not live without Drew; I could not live with myself. She was shocked. Such a reaction, she said, was rather 'extreme'. I needed to see a psychiatrist as soon as possible. I was insulted: it was not as if I had just lost a pet.

Three weeks later I had my initial appraisal. I cried more than I talked. At the end of the hour the head doctor said that I had been left in the lurch. Drew enabled me to control the other conflicts in my life – parents, career, sexuality – which now threatened to overwhelm me. I was clinging to my grief because there was nothing else to hold on to; I was afraid of losing Drew if I lost the pain. There was the distinct possibility that I would kill myself and he understood why. Therapy could help, although it would be a painful process. I should think about it and let him know my decision the following week.

The consulting rooms were in East Finchley. I walked over the hill to St Pancras and Islington Cemetery, the site of Drew's cremation. A freezing wind moaned among the gardens of stone. I cried when the chimney came into view. The vast necropolis was deserted at lunchtime on Saturday. The crematorium, however, was open. I had to see inside. Clean lines, pale wood, fresh flowers: the stage was set for the next curtain call. I should have been there for Drew's.

Perhaps, if I had witnessed his coffin rolling towards the oven, it would have brought his death home to me. As it was, I felt that half of me was missing. I would stretch out my arm on the sofa to where Drew used to sit but meet thin air not warm flesh. Trailing round Marks & Spencer, shopping for one, I saw some avocados and realised he would never make guacamole again. Every day was the anniversary of something: I relived the events of the previous year blow by blow. Fresh memories of old horrors surfaced daily. The eighth of May was a bank holiday: somebody else's chemotherapy was being delayed while the nation celebrated the fiftieth anniversary of VE Day. I watched the fly-past from Drew's bedroom window. It was rounded off by the Red Arrows, trailing smoking streamers of red, white and blue. Lest we forget . . . It was important to remember.

I saw the psychiatrist assigned to me five times. Each session in the north London basement was worse than the last. He told me straight away that short-term grief counselling would not be of much use: long-term analysis was my only way out. In other words, I was a basket-case. I had always been sceptical about psychiatry: its practitioners were just post-structuralists who had swapped their lecture rooms for consulting rooms. Alex had been in and out of therapy for years. He treated it like a fashion accessory. A good shrink, according to him, was as essential as a good personal trainer. It never seemed to make him a happier or better person. As my mother said, chat changed nothing.

The psychiatrist asked questions but would not answer any. He cut the conversation as soon as forty-five minutes had elapsed. It was infuriating. I tried to use my anger to control my tears. He accused me of attempting to blackmail him: 'You're giving me an ultimatum: cure me or I'll kill myself.' He was wrong: I wanted to kill *him*. His theory was that I was furious with Drew and wished to get back at him by ending my own life. I was filled with rage, it was true, but the suggestion that I was angry with Drew horrified me. Of all the things I felt for him, fury was not one of them. It was not Drew's fault that he died – and it was not mine either.

I wanted to die to stop the pain. The psychiatrist implied that I had got Drew's death out of all proportion. We had been together less than two years: as my life went on its impact would diminish. In other words, it was not that important. The fact that the love of my life had endured a slow, agonising death seemed not to register with the man. I considered it highly irresponsible to belittle Drew's memory, to blame other factors for the way I felt. Commit suicide over a dead boyfriend? I must be mad.

I did not trust him. I longed to talk about what I had done – after all, no one else wanted to know – and I needed to explore why, although I was convinced I had done the right thing, I still felt a residual guilt. However, I saw him as a hired listener rather than a secret-sharer, and he soon proved his unsuitability by writing to my GP. She showed me the letter when I went to ask for some Temazepam. Mark Sanderson was 'actively suicidal', 'becoming increasingly withdrawn' and 'pathologically mourning'. He was right, up to a point, but the next sentence made me flush: 'I hope it will not be necessary to hospitalise him during the breaks in therapy.' I was embarrassed. Drugged up and drooling in a strait-jacket? Me? I laughed and said the man viewed me as a gold mine. I was depressed, but not that depressed. The last thing I needed was more time in hospital.

I had assumed that what was said in the consulting room would be confidential, so was glad I had not laid myself open to prosecution. I wrote him a letter explaining that I no longer wished to proceed with the therapy. Honesty was not the best policy. Conflict made life interesting. It was foolish to think it could all be talked away. What was the point of making decisions, favouring duty or desire, doing the right or wrong thing, if there was nothing at stake?

The problem was that I felt I had nothing left to lose. My career had crumbled and the flat meant little without Drew. One morning the paper-boy rang the doorbell: I had left the key in the lock all night. No one had entered my room: at least one nightmare had not come true. Perhaps I should move into my grandmother's house? It was empty. My parents were not enthusiastic. 'Your life is in London now,' said my father. 'Besides, your mother wants to sell it.' I could not countenance moving into another rented flat and there was no way I would return to Shakespeare Walk.

I turned my back on the world. When two media recruitment agencies failed to get me a single interview I gave up. *Monopolies of Loss* by Adam Mars-Jones meant a lot more on a second reading. I spent my days doing old crosswords from the *Listener*. The Crossword Club published one I had compiled under a pseudonym. 'Walkabout' was based on a dictionary of aboriginal words that Drew had given me. I dedicated it to Drew. I re-watched films that we had seen together, and even found myself, at odd moments, laughing like Drew. He had a wicked, dirty snicker. I turned down invitations to dinner or the cinema and stayed on the sofa with the curtains closed. Some days the only person I spoke to was Drew. I compiled a photo album of the two of us. It took a week but represented real progress: I could not bring myself to play the video of the cruise. If one word summed up this period it was 'withdrew'. The meaning of words was the only meaning I could find.

In the end boredom got me back on my feet. I returned to the gym with trepidation. It was like starting all over again. I was so unfit I nearly fainted on the exercise bike. Pedalling furiously and getting nowhere: the story of my life. Grief could ambush me at any time. I would be on the rowing machine with tears rolling down my face but if anyone did notice they must have assumed it was sweat. I watched the men changing in the locker rooms and marvelled at their physical health. I had to bite my tongue whenever one of them returned, half-cooked, from a sun-bed. I could have asked if they had ever seen someone dying of skin cancer but they would only have told me to fuck off. I could have assured them they would be just as good-looking without a tan but they would only have told me to fuck off. I had become what I hated most: a lonely old queen. Someone to be ignored like the dregs of the sauna in Nice.

However, the fact that gays and straights still shared locker rooms proved that heterosexual men did not have everything their own way. Heterosexual men moved in a different way to gay men. It was their easy self-confidence that made them so attractive. It was a straight world and they knew it. They were just as aware of their own sex, spent just as much time studying prospective rivals as potential partners, but did not go to bed with other men. Not often, anyway. They behaved as society expected them to behave because that was how they were programmed: they did not have to be continually on their guard, they did not need to think about what they said and did all the time. It was an enviable existence. Their basic instincts and inherited power produced a natural arrogance that made them irresistible to many gays. Any demonstration of sensitivity merely increased the attraction. There was nothing more erotic than watching a proud father pushing his new-born baby down the street. 'Real' men, however, only had sex with real women. There was no point in lusting after straight guys. You might as well fall in love with a ghost.

On the other hand, some of them liked the attention. One

quiet Friday afternoon I coincided with a boy I called the Armani Model in the steam room. He treated the central aisle of the changing room like a catwalk. He would saunter down it stark naked, a white towel in his hand, staring at himself in the mirrors. He would have been even more beautiful had he been less self-aware. I had caught his eye a thousand times. He liked to know he was being watched. There was no one else in the steam room. He started stroking his cock. I did not need telling twice. It was all over in a couple of minutes. I was still on my knees when, in pure Essex, he said: 'You fucking poof.' Some fantasies did come true.

No one would employ me so I had to employ myself. Writing was the one thing I could do pretty well. I would write myself out of the mess. Elaine and I worked on a sitcom together. 'EBF', erotic best friends, was a comedy about a gay man and a straight woman who shared a flat. Nothing came of it but, as *Will and Grace* proved years later, it was not such a bad idea. When Brian became the Books Editor of *Time Out*, the former Film Editor sent me a biography of Terence Rattigan and suggested I start reviewing for the magazine again. It was the spur I needed. I exhumed *Snow Hill* and decided to rework it from scratch.

The wheel of fortune seemed to have turned full circle. Macmillan decided to publish a revised edition of the *Inspector Morse* book to tie in with the return of the series. I was commissioned to write one new chapter of 3,000 words. The rattling Tube to Harrow-on-the-Hill sent me back to 1992: the local Territorial Army Volunteer Reserve centre had been converted into an Oxford police station for 'The Way Through the Woods'. It was as if nothing had changed. Familiar faces were organising the chaos; John Thaw and Kevin Whately looked just the same. They even appeared pleased to see me.

The day before I had noticed the imprint of Drew's briefcase on the carpet of his bedroom floor. He had kept it beside the chest of drawers. It was now almost a year since his parents had taken it back to Australia. My impressions of the time were just as fresh. I interviewed Thaw in his Winnebago during the lunch break. As usual, he was smoking the cigarettes that would eventually kill him. We continued chatting after I had turned off the tape-recorder and before I knew it I was telling him all about Drew and how I had watched 'Masonic Mysteries' on the day he died. I did not cry but my voice quavered. Drew was not at the end of a telephone in Jericho now. 'There's no time-limit on grief,' said Thaw. 'Take as long as you need. Some people need only weeks to recover, others months or years. It's different for everyone.' Later in the afternoon, while I was sitting in a corner, watching Sergeant Lewis walk down the corridor into Morse's office, Thaw came over and handed me a note. It was a street map of Oxford city centre: 'To Mark, with all best wishes from John. I'm glad old E. Morse helped a little.' I dedicated the new edition to Drew.

Geoff, who replaced Brian as Film Editor, introduced me to Ed Buscombe at the British Film Institute. A new series of monographs called Modern Classics was being planned to accompany the successful BFI Classics – short, personal studies of individual films. Melvyn Bragg, for example, had cracked Ingmar Bergman's *The Seventh Seal* and Salman Rushdie had followed the yellow brick road to *The Wizard of Oz*. I proposed 20,000 words on *Don't Look Now*.

Nic Roeg's tale of death in Venice had long been in my list of top ten films. However, it was only when I came to study it in detail that I realised that the Gothic thriller was actually a profound exploration of grief. The drowning of their young daughter plunges the Baxters into a welter of anger, fear and guilt. Laura Baxter, played by Julie Christie, cannot accept that her child has gone. A blind Scottish medium claims to have seen Christine and offers to get in touch with her; John Baxter, played by Donald Sutherland, has no truck with such 'mumbo-jumbo' but keeps catching sight of a red-coated figure that bears a striking resemblance to Christine. The most shocking line in the ghost story comes when John loses patience with his 'crazy' wife and tells her that Christine is 'dead – dead, dead, dead, dead, dead!'

The act of writing the book was, inevitably, a painful process. However, it provided only a partial catharsis. I could express my feelings of loss but I could only flirt with the truth: 'Guilt is often felt following bereavement – even if not directly responsible, your inability to prevent the death still rankles – and the fact that you go on living while your loved one does not can be enough to create a sense of being in the wrong.' The line 'when someone you love dies in your arms it changes you for ever' became 'when someone you love dies a part of you dies with them'. I was pleased with the first version but rewrote it because, in one way, it was not true.

Auden, as usual, had said it all before. I chose four lines from 'Twelve Songs' as an epigraph:

> Behind the corpse in the reservoir, behind the ghost on
> the links,
> Behind the lady who dances and the man who madly
> drinks,
> Under the look of fatigue, the attack of migraine and the
> sigh
> There is always another story, there is more than meets
> the eye.

I dedicated the book to Drew and sent a copy to his parents. I also sent copies to John Thaw and Germaine Greer. It was as if I wanted to let them know that I was still here – and Drew was not. We had obeyed Germaine's injunction: we had stayed together for as long as we could. Her reply was typically perceptive: 'There is nothing I can say to help you at this time – I know that being told "you will get over it" is the most heartbreaking thing.'

The books were cries for help but I was directing them at the wrong people. I could not be myself with my family so I was bothering virtual strangers. It was unprofessional. The fact that I no longer made any distinction between public and private was another sign that I was losing my grip.

I was not the only one. The editor of *GQ* magazine killed himself in his Islington flat. The man next door tried to gas himself in his van. The whole world seemed to be mad. Each week I forced myself to reply to a Talking Heart ad in *Time Out*. Each call was supposed to represent a positive step but the men I met were just as wounded. The grounded airline pilot; the hysterical researcher from the BBC; the vicar who suffered a crisis of conscience and cancelled the third date: they were all equally miserable. The most promising meeting came to an abrupt end when the ex-wife of the company director received a telephone call informing her William was moving to Islington to live with a man – and planned to take the children with him. The woman had to be rushed into hospital to have her stomach pumped out. I felt nothing for these potential lovers: they were competing with a ghost. I could not imagine being intimate with anyone ever again. It was not in my nature to settle for second best. The sex was meaningless. I saw no reason to refuse. Each disaster proved I was better off alone.

I became an uncle – and a godfather. I thought Linda and Craig were mad to consider bringing a child into this world. I fixated on the worry it would create, not the love. However, when Linda first placed the tiny bundle, sleeping hotly, in my arms I felt a rush of emotion. Curtis was the son I would never have. Drew had often joked about us having a baby. I knew instinctively and without question that I would do anything to protect my nephew. Perhaps that was why I was attracted to novice fathers: they could not help exuding both strength and tenderness.

I expected to be struck by a thunderbolt during the chris-
tening service when I renounced the devil and all his works.
The vicar's mention of 'dear, departed ones' moved me
deeply – although he was referring to our grandparents, not
my boyfriend. There was so much love in our family yet it
would be irrelevant if I could not be myself. I was sick of
having to censor my conversation, of telling little white lies.
It was one thing to spare a person's feelings, quite another to
protect their prejudices. I carried on smiling through hell.

There were times, on long walks beside the Lune, when I
toyed with telling my father the truth. He had refused to
allow the bank to foreclose on me – my overdraft had con-
tinued to grow – and written me a cheque for £25,000.
Would he have done so if he had known his son was gay?
I doubted it. His first response to the Archbishop of
Canterbury's midnight blessing on New Year's Eve was 'the
Bible says nothing about homosexual and women priests'.

The tears dried up as my depression deepened. I felt alone
even when I had company – and I soon had more than ever
before. Pascal and Marta needed somewhere to live while
builders turned a Bethnal Green loft into their dream home.
I needed to pay the rent. It would only be for six weeks. To
begin with it was a relief to have someone to care for again.
I did the laundry, collected their dry-cleaning, and generally
kept the flat running as smoothly as possible. The couple
were like visitors from another planet. Marta could not
choose between a job that paid £80,000 and another that

paid £100,000. Their hectic social life highlighted my reclusion.

Nor could I work on *Snow Hill* while lodgers were around. My agent had approved the revised treatment and told me to go ahead and write the first six chapters. I came up with a good opening sentence: 'I went to my funeral this morning.' As the computer was in their – Drew's – room I had to break off as soon as I heard the key in the lock, even if the words were flowing, and this added to my frustration. There was no space to put the machine anywhere else. It cannot have been easy for Pascal and Marta to live with such an awkward, uptight landlord. Our stress levels soared. My gums started bleeding. I had a permanent cold and succumbed to laryngitis and bronchitis. Illness shortened my temper. We rowed. They accused me of loving not them but their money.

It was Alex, however, who nearly ended our friendship. He continued to climb the property ladder as his earning curve steepened. The sale of his latest flat in Bayswater was about to go through but he and Guy had yet to find a place to buy together. Could they stay in Packington Street for a while? A few days after I agreed Guy was rushed into the Chelsea and Westminster hospital with pneumonia. Aids was diagnosed. Alex was furious: Guy had not told him he was HIV-positive. The Frenchman said he had not known. Alex refused to take a test: 'I've enough to deal with as it is.' I did not press him because I was worried what the result would be. I did not want to lose Alex as well.

Pascal and Marta were reluctant to leave: the builders, of course, were behind schedule. They had hoped to stay a bit longer. I explained that Guy, who had recovered surprisingly quickly, was about to be released from hospital. He and Alex were homeless. I could not see my best friend on the street. His boyfriend was dying . . . They went. It was all my fault.

Alex and I were both trapped. While it seemed he would now, finally, learn what Drew and I had been through I had no desire to go through it again. Neither of us had any choice. Alex, however, was expert at getting away with things and in a physical sense he did get away. His job involved frequent trips abroad so while he flew to Bombay or Washington or Madrid I was at home with Guy. His boyfriend was typically French: his hauteur masked a hankering for the gutter. His striking features stemmed partly from their unnatural symmetry: his face had been rebuilt after a motorcycle accident when he was sixteen. His nose, as you would discover to your cost during a clumsy kiss, was made of stainless steel. Alex teased him about his heavy build and, unaware of the terrible irony, called him Lumpy.

They lived with me for three months. Guy kept his pills in the same kitchen cupboard as Drew. The constant naps, the frequent telephone enquiries from friends, the awkward moments in television soaps, the sudden panics as other symptoms occurred, all brought back new details of Drew's ordeal. On a shopping trip to Marks & Spencer we had to stop – 'Now!' – for a rest. I bought a bottle of mineral water but wished it were vodka. The same thing had happened with Drew. The wheel of fortune had turned into a vicious circle.

Alex dealt with the situation in his own way: he went to sex joints, rubber clubs and leather bars. When he finally summoned up the courage to have an Aids test the result, fifteen minutes later, was negative. 'And does watching skinheads drink each other's piss make you feel better?' 'Sort of. It's not something you see every day. You're such a suburban puritan – have some more coke and shut up.' It was a reward for providing yet another alibi.

Cocaine did help. At first I experienced the same euphoria and urge to talk as everyone else. However, I soon came to love the drug for other reasons. It did not make me feel happy, it made me feel nothing at all and as such provided a means of escape. It placed me in a bubble, buoyed me up, let me float off while those around me chattered on. Cocaine allowed me to lose control in a controlled way. The ritual of crushing the lumps and chopping the powder was half the fun and I prolonged it for as long as I could, enjoying the mixture of anticipation and dread. The white lines promised pleasure yet proved the weakness of my will. I was careful not to meet my eyes in the mirror. I disapproved of drugs and those who took them.

To begin with I could not afford to buy cocaine. I did not really need to, though: there was a lot of it about. Most people liked to share. I would follow them back to their Georgian townhouse, Barbican penthouse or Whitehall flat and wonder what made them do it. They had lovers, careers and beautiful homes but something must have been missing. Hours disappeared in seconds. I would take my leave as it began to get light and walk home through the empty streets.

Reality dawned along with the day. The feeble birdsong echoed my nihilism.

Self-disgust was the worst of the side-effects. I was used to feeling ill and exhausted. I had a migraine most days anyway. Drew had refused to have anything to do with recreational drugs, and I had not taken them while we were together, but now I was using his death as an excuse to get wrecked. I had reached the point where I did not care what happened to me. I was on my way out. It was time for a last hurrah.

I had never been a party animal as I found it difficult to let myself go. Cocaine, on the other hand, unleashed the animal in me. I performed my party trick – sucking myself off – or stripped and sucked off other people. Cocaine may have shrunk the penis but an erection was usually possible. Besides, the magic dust turned heterosexuals gay for the night, and straight men tasted better. I felt no shame. Such depravity was an excellent way of releasing frustration – for them and for me. They had an orgasm and, if I could not speak the truth – 'I killed my boyfriend' – then at least I could reveal my true self: this poor, bare, fucked-up animal was me.

I was not interested in other drugs. If I had a line of cocaine I immediately wanted another but my addiction would only last for the night. I might end up snorting a gram then not take any more for three months. Alex, though, would put anything up his nose. At one of his soirées the white powder turned out to be ketamine, a horse tranquilliser known as 'Special K'. My vision blurred, my speech slurred and I became totally incapacitated. I was hurtling backwards down a dark tunnel. Panic and paralysis was an infernal combination. 'Don't worry,' said Alex. 'It won't last for ever. You're in a K-hole, enjoy it.' I lay on the floor and looked up at the giggling idiots swaying around me. A ring of gargoyles: this would be the last thing anyone who over-dosed in a club would see. It was a ridiculous way to die.

One night, after another of Alex's parties, I determined how I *would* die. The builders had finally admitted that a new roof was the only way to stop the leak in Drew's room. Once the scaffolding had been erected they discovered the men who had recently replaced the slates next door had not only dumped the debris on the roof above my head but defecated – more than once – in the gutter. I told them I was used to being shat on.

Snow Hill – Alex had not failed to point out the chemical irony – had only received 'rave rejections', each one contra-dicting the last: 'Too quaint,' said Bantam; 'Too hardboiled,' said Macmillan. Carole Blake suggested that, after five years, it was time to call it a day and go our separate ways. She earned her living obtaining advances; I spent my life making retreats. The disappointment, although expected, was crush-ing. All that work, often in the most difficult of circumstances, had come to nothing.

It had been a heavy Saturday night in Hammersmith: in the end I had lost all power of suction. I was finished. Cocaine destroyed the soul as well as the septum. It was a false friend that provided only illusory support. I held hands with Steven in the cab but, just as he had always done, he refused to sleep with me. Begging made no difference. The Asian driver lis-tened in silence. No closure there then. I watched the cab turn out of Packington Street. There was a glorious sunrise. Now was as good a time as any – I went straight upstairs, flung off my clothes, opened the window and clambered out on to the scaffolding. The rungs of the ladder felt as though they were slicing my feet in half.

I had never been on the roof before. I stood on the brink. The view was spectacular. There was the Euston tower, the Telecom tower, Centrepoint and the Old Bailey. The statue of Justice shimmered in the sun.

'Way to go!' Seventy feet below, a young clubber, homeward bound, waved and carried on down the road. He did not look back. He was probably on drugs himself. I suddenly felt stupid and cold. I retreated to Drew's bed. If I was going to commit suicide then I must plan it properly and stop pussyfooting around.

In 1995 I told Drew's father that I intended to make a will. Would he mind if I were to leave instructions for my ashes to be sprinkled over Drew's grave? He wrote back to say he was sure I would prefer them to be buried alongside Drew's. He gave me the plot number and the address of the cemetery. I shed tears of gratitude. Now, two years on, I planned to visit our final resting place, make peace with his family, go on a pilgrimage to Coochiemudlo Island then jump off Sydney Harbour Bridge at night. No one would notice another drop in the ocean.

The flat seemed much larger when Alex and Guy had gone. It was a relief to be alone again. The peace and quiet made me feel Drew's absence all the more. He still received junk mail and the odd telephone call. Why had Mr Morgan not filed a VAT return? Would he care to join BUPA?

Sex did not fill the emotional void yet I still went after it. I was desperate for some kind of connection. I made passes at total strangers: waiters, the boys in Oddbins (who blushed), even my new Marxist window-cleaner. He responded by lending me his copy of Noam Chomsky's *Manufacturing Consent*. Sex was a service industry too but satisfaction was not guaranteed. The whore who arrived late one Friday night was from New Zealand, not Australia as I had requested. 'Reef' said he lived in Old Compton Street, above the minicab office: 'It's very convenient.' He laughed when I asked if he was a student. Did he want to be an actor? 'No, no, no. This is what I do.' He was a disco-bunny, bursting with youth rather than beauty. His gym-toned musculature did not suit him: it was as if he had slipped on a special, body-hugging T-shirt that gave him instant latex pecs and abs. He was out of his head on ketamine: I gave him the £150 anyway. I felt sorry for him although, in the circumstances, I should have saved the pity for myself. Paying for cock showed how low I had sunk. I was Reef's fifth client of the evening. It took him ages to come. He was back on his mobile as he went down the stairs.

I had returned to the *Sunday Times* in April 1997. It was the only way I could earn a decent amount of money: first-class air tickets to Australia did not come cheap. If I was going to go out, I was going to do so in style. Subbing shifts were generally available on the television pages because the work was so vile. Some people quit before they had even completed their first week's training. The hourly rate was about to be increased as well: I no longer needed a lodger. All I had to do now was knuckle under and settle my debts.

It took almost a year. However, having an end in sight lent me staying power. In the aftermath of Drew's death I had continually set myself artificial deadlines: my birthday, the publication of *The Times* crossword No. 20,000, the release of Peter Greenaway's *The Pillow Book*. Parcelling out time made survival seem easier, less daunting. The sale of Shakespeare Walk enabled me to pay back most of my friends; my parents, as next-of-kin, would receive the benefits of the life assurance policy that I had taken out with the mortgage. The bank manager had told me insurers worked on the assumption that no one planned a suicide more than two years ahead.

As I approached the door of the 12.15 Qantas flight to Sydney I found myself alongside one of the personal trainers from the gym. He was going home. He turned right and I turned left. When the stewardess saw my boarding pass she gave a mock bow: 'It's God himself!' She led me to seat 1A.

The novelty of lobster and Krug at 33,000 feet soon wore off. Even at 600mph, the jumbo was still hours away from Sydney when it finally crossed the west coast of Australia. I began to realise just how far Drew had come.

The harbour view seemed totally familiar and utterly strange. I wandered along the waterfront from Bennelong Point to The Rocks, the bridge never out of my sight or my mind. I would only set foot on it when my farewell tour was complete. Whereas most British men were neither good-looking nor bad, simply lurking in-between, Australian men appeared to have been either blessed with beauty or bashed about the head with the ugly stick. And when they did look you right in the eye, it was impossible to tell if they were going to kiss you or kill you.

Alex had been to Sydney the year before. He had called on his mobile as he and a fellow coke-fiend had sailed past the Opera House sipping champagne: 'Glad you're not here!' He had no idea of my plan – I had not told anyone – but he managed to surprise me when, learning of my trip, he remarked: 'Well, you've always done what you wanted. That's what I admire about you. I don't know anyone else who has.' Hence, no doubt, why I was now in such a mess.

Alex gave me Greg's telephone numbers. His former lodger had returned home in 1994 and did not remember me. He remembered Drew, though. I told him what had happened. He invited me to an Oscar Night party he and his partner were hosting that evening in Surry Hills. It was reassuring to be surrounded by Australian voices. I met a blond surfer who came back to my hotel. His buttocks were the only part of him that was not nut-brown. They seemed to glow in the dark.

I was supposed to stay for a week on Coochiemudlo Island. Jan and Ron had built the house themselves to a design intended to take maximum advantage of the cross breezes in

Moreton Bay. This, apparently, explained the internal window in the bathroom which was unglazed and uncurtained. Anyone who walked by could see you on the dunny – which, due to the water shortage, was only to be flushed after 'number twos'. Two fat corgis, who looked like an old lesbian couple, waddled around the place sniffing after Shazz, the second house guest. We were expected to share a room. I knew it was not going to work out.

Coochie was a patch of paradise. The beaches, during the week, were deserted. The curlews and kookaburras made an exotic change from copulating pigeons. It was a far cry from Islington, and I could see why Drew had loved it, but he was not here now. I had hoped his presence might be felt in his favourite place. My disappointment and despair exploded at the drunken barbecue that evening. Drew had been a different person to all of us: we each thought we knew the real Drew. He was the only thing we had in common. I left the table and ran down to the water's edge unable to hold back the tears any longer. The Milky Way wheeled above. I had never seen so many stars. I was trapped again. Shazz whimpered in her sleep. The air-conditioning unit did not work. The mozzies were a pain. The next day I checked back into the Sheraton in Brisbane.

I had dinner with Drew's brother twice – once with Jenny, his new girlfriend, and once with Jan, his ex. I wondered what he looked like with his pony-tail undone. David also worked in computers. He showed signs of stoicism rather than grief; I was touched by his fierce loyalty to his parents. Jan showed me round the house in Swan Terrace that Drew had shared with his brother. She was about to move out to make room for her successor. I sometimes ventured into the parallel universe where Drew had been miraculously cured. Would we have lived happily ever after or drifted apart, had affairs, split up — amicably or acrimoniously — and gone our separate ways? I was sure that we would have stayed together.

The side of the house was streaked with fruit bat shit. Drew had stood in this garden, beneath this umbrella tree, on the eve of his trip to England. He had heard those windchimes tinkling. He was at peace. It was all right for him: my pain just went on and on. I was still living with the consequences of that hot night in his room. Every day I answered the same question. Yes, you did the right thing. I had to be strong for just a little longer. The agony would soon be over.

I reached the grave on Palm Sunday. It was the best-kept plot in the cemetery. The fresh white paint glowed in the late afternoon sun. It was a picturesque spot, surrounded by trees, although the tranquillity was regularly shattered by jets taking off from the nearby airport. I placed the two red roses on top of the concrete tomb. My mother had asked me to buy one for her. It represented a reconciliation of sorts.

The decision to bury the ashes in 1994 had seemed a halfway gesture, a compromise between ecology and eternity. Drew had not got clean away. However, the grave provided a focus for his family's grief. The brass plaque hinted at anger:

December 1964 Mossman – London July 1994

DREW FRANCIS MORGAN

Beloved son, brother, brother-in-law, uncle

Loved and cherished in life

and through all eternity

'Take care of you for us'

'London' was my sole acknowledgement. The fact that there were no dates was odd. Had they suspected something after all? My blood turned to lead.

A wattle tree grew beside the grave. A plant with yellow flowers – which Jack later told me was an allamanda – had wound itself round its branches. As I dried my eyes I saw one of the twigs come to life. It was a snake. Its black eyes glittered. I was not going to move: it had taken me four years to get here. This was my grave too. The perfect place to die. The worm slithered away.

The sun sank behind the distant mountains. Strange birds called to each other. Another jumbo lumbered into the sky. Drew was not here just as he was not on Coochiemudlo or at Wraysbury. He was in my head and in my heart, nowhere else. There was no point in looking for him: he had been with me all the time.

The Morgans lived only a short walk away. His father showed me round the house while his mother cooked dinner. Drew's room was as small as mine in Packington Street. With more window than wall, it felt as though you were outside rather than in. I understood now why he had been able to sleep anywhere. Jasper, his pet cockatoo, still screeched and talked to herself in the yard. They had thought she was male until she laid an egg. The warning her young owner had mis-spelled in white paint remained on the side of the cage: 'Jasper lives here! SRATCH.'

We drank a couple of bottles of Yellowglen fizz with the roast lamb. There were lychees and ice-cream to follow. Drew had introduced me to the fruit. It was his favourite. The humid air was full of things unsaid. Lizards scuttled across wooden walls covered in photographs of Drew. His early days had been so different from my own. It was hard to believe that this little boy, grinning on the other side of the world, had become the love of my life.

It was pleasant to walk along the Esplanade, when the tide hid the mangrove swamp, but there was nothing else to do in Cairns. I had a day out with Jack and Aileen. They showed me the hospital in Mossman where Drew was born and the house in Crawford Street to which he went home. We had lunch in Port Douglas and drove back through the sugarcane fields, occasionally stopping to admire the views of the Coral Sea. I took Debbie, Simon and Carly to Kuranda, a mountain refuge for hippies. We went up by steam train and down by cable car, skimming the canopy of the ancient rainforest. 'It's like riding a magic green carpet,' said Carly. We wrote to each other every couple of months now. I had become an agony uncle, dispensing advice on boys and books. Her energy and optimism, hurled on to the page, made me feel decrepit.

Although the scenery was stunning I could not take my eyes off Debbie. The resemblance to Drew had grown. Her facial expressions and mannerisms were uncannily similar. The Morgans seemed to accept that I had loved Drew deeply, that he was still a big part of my life. I knew they were seeing me for his sake as well as mine.

I could see the yellow flowers on the wattle tree as the plane banked after take-off. I had been back to the grave on a couple of occasions. The last time, as I was leaving, a double rainbow appeared. Debbie or Simon must have had a word with their colleagues because, as we approached Sydney, I was invited into the cockpit. The view was spectacular: Westminster Bridge and the Golden Gate Bridge did not afford a better panorama. The harbour, and the scene of my death, lay straight ahead.

The sheer scale of the bridge was intimidating. On Good Friday I went on a tour of the harbour. The ferry sailed round Pinchgut Island, otherwise known as Fort Denison – where the corpse of convict Francis Morgan had hung in chains – and passed beneath the massive span. So this is where I would end up. I knew the water would feel like concrete.

I ordered my last supper from room service and wrote a letter to my parents: 'I tried. Sorry.' They would be all right. They had a grandson to take care of now. I left a note of apology to the hotel manager and asked him to telephone Drew's parents and my own. Jack would see that my final request was fulfilled. Aileen would receive the crucifix round my neck after all.

Ninety minutes later I was back in the room. I was also soaked to the skin – but not from sea-water. As I stood in the middle of the bridge, cursing my stupidity, the heavens had opened. I really was out of my mind. I was hardly the first person to have considered jumping to my death. The walkway was a caged tunnel: you could not even jump into the endless stream of traffic. You could either advance to the north side or retreat to the south. The lightning made every rivet in the cat's-cradle of girders stand out. I was such an idiot. I trailed back through the storm, just one more pathetic Pom skidding across the marble foyer. If I had known about the Gap, where suicidal Sydneysiders leapt off sandstone cliffs at the end of Old South Head Road, I would have got into a cab there and then. However, ignorance saved me again.

It was only when I knew I had failed that the fear and panic had returned. The closer I had got to the bridge the calmer I had become. Back in London, I felt no fear as I washed down forty Sevredol with the last of the Dom Pérignon Drew had bought in Paris. Surely 2,000mg would do? I had no desire to spend the rest of my life sub-editing television schedules in a windowless hangar. I had become increasingly dislocated as the week had dragged on. I expected each flagstone to swing open and swallow me up. Nothing would remove the metallic taste in my mouth. Out on the terrace a single iris, planted by Drew, was in bloom.

Vertigo was playing for the third time that evening. James Stewart pulled Kim Novak out of the bay once again. You could not bring people back from the dead: you could only go on to join them.

The stench in the hot room was horrendous. At some stage I had thrown up. I could only keep awake for a few seconds. Each time I emerged into consciousness I crawled a bit further along the floor. So this is what it felt like: I was dying. Third time lucky. I had a raging thirst. I gagged again. The carpet pressed into my face. It felt like wire-wool.

It was Monday morning before I finally managed to get to my feet. Sunday was a gap in the calendar. 'Migraine' did not begin to describe the headache. I could not stop shivering. My eyes were bloodshot, my lips were cracked, my joints were stiff and my muscles were cramped. I felt sick, dizzy and thirsty. I drank lots of water, took a couple of painkillers and forced myself to eat a banana. I nearly brought it back up as I cleared away the vomit. Leo had said this would happen. I had failed yet again. I went to bed. Drew was not ready for me, that was it. I suppose that meant I had to go on.

12

ONWARDS

A rthur, the old soldier from downstairs, died on 23 April. It was on the same day, five years earlier, that Drew had called to say, 'Let's get a place together.' Elsie came up to tell me the bad news. 'We were married fifty years, four months, ten days and six hours. The funeral's next Friday. If I get through this week I'll be all right. Then we can get on with our lives.' Such resilience filled me with shame. Elsie was in no doubt that you had to press on.

The morphine sulphate had been over a year past its use-by date. Perhaps it had lost its potency. Perhaps I had not taken enough. Perhaps Drew had saved me. After the suicide attempt I dreamed about him frequently. He was in the garden, standing at the bottom of the spiral staircase. I was at the top. I told him: 'I don't see much of you nowadays' . . . I stretched to kiss him. He moved away. I stretched to kiss him. He moved away. Was he angry with me? . . . Another night he was simply waving goodbye. Most mornings I woke up crying. Drew lived on in my mind: if I died, so would the memories.

Your life can change at any moment, whether you want it to or not. Brian handed me the letter. It had been sent to *Time Out* and was marked 'Private & Confidential':

> Dear Mark Sanderson, I've been enjoying your reviews in *Time Out* and I wondered if you'd like to do some for me here too? Do please give me a ring.

It was from the Literary Editor of the *Evening Standard*. Was it a cruel joke? I had replied to dozens of job applications in the *Guardian* and yet not one trade publication or regional rag, not a single specialist title or glossy magazine, had even short-listed me for an interview. Now a well-known newspaper was offering me work. Was it true? My hand shook as I keyed in the number of the direct line.

The boost to my ego could not have come at a better time. Someone had faith in me. I continued to review books for *Time Out* as well as the *Standard* even though the latter paid six times as much per review. I stuck it out at the *Sunday Times* for another nine months. Two weeks after I quit, the *Sunday Telegraph* telephoned. They were looking for someone to write a column called 'The Literary Life'. The present incumbent, Alain de Botton, was moving on to greater things. Was

I interested? It took me all of twenty-four hours to decide that I could do it.

'The Literary Life' was not a gossip column. It featured items of general interest to the general reader: who was writing what rather than who was sleeping with whom. I found most of my stories at book launches, publishing parties and award ceremonies. They were often held in gentlemen's clubs, foreign embassies or parliamentary chambers: rooms I had never expected to enter. One launch was held in the Great Hall at Bart's. It was the first time I had been back to the hospital. We had both been reprieved. Free booze loosened the ties and tongues of authors, agents and publicists. The column was an ideal chance to get back into the world of books. Soon other literary editors invited me to contribute to their pages. The impossible had happened: I was making a living by doing something I loved.

The bookshelves in the living room slowly refilled, and the videos went back into storage. Douglas Adams now stood between Peter Ackroyd and Martin Amis. Drew would have been pleased. However, I still found myself looking for books that were sold years ago: ghost literature. Parts of my mind were arrested in time, imprisoned in 1994.

One morning, just before I left the *Sunday Times*, I entered the office to see Drew sitting at one of the terminals. There must have been a computer problem which he was trying to sort out. I was about to put my hand on his shoulder, had already opened my mouth to say, 'What are you doing here?', when reality hit me. I dropped my arm, shut my mouth and hurried to my desk. When I sat down I was shaking. The fact that I could deceive myself, after five years, was almost as shocking as the resemblance. It had to be Drew: everything about the man was the same. It took me all morning to catch his eye: not a flicker of recognition. He must have thought I fancied him: in one way, of course, I did. I never saw the guy from systems again.

I am haunted by Drew; I expect I always will be. It is not an unusual phenomenon. Apart from Ruth Brandon's 1996 novel, *The Uncertainty Principle*, I have avoided reading about the subject. However, when you open a book, as when you open a door, you do not know who or what you are going to meet. The title piece in *Heavy Water and Other Stories* by Martin Amis, which I reviewed for *Time Out* in 1998, put me back on the cross-channel ferry with Drew; *The Snakebite Survivors' Club* by Jeremy Seal, which I reviewed for the *Standard* in 1999, took me back to the cemetery in Cairns. The first herpetologist to bag a taipan, one of the world's deadliest snakes, was bitten as he did so. He is buried in the same boneyard as Drew. I made a mental note to run the next time I saw a twig come alive.

'Death is nothing at all,' wrote Henry Scott-Holland. 'I have only slipped away into the next room. I am I and you are you; whatever we were to each other that we are still.' Death is not 'the next room', it is the same room. It is all around us. Not thinking about it does not make it go away. Drew is in my memory even when I am not remembering him. What happened on 16 July 1994 slowly poisoned me. I was haunted by the way Drew died. Guilt thrives on lies and secrecy. To make a clean break I needed to come clean.

In May 2000 I returned to Australia to report on the Sydney Writers' Festival. Many of the events were held in the waterfront premises of the Sydney Theatre Company off Hickson Road. One evening, on my way back to the hotel, I stopped at Dawes Point. The bridge loomed overhead. I realised that I was glad I had not jumped. I had heard a lot of talk about epiphanies, issues and unresolved conflicts in the past few days. Drew's death was the defining moment of my life. It proved that I could put another person's well-being before my own. There was nothing unusual about a young man dying of cancer, but the circumstances surrounding Drew's demise were extraordinary. I knew, no matter how many times people assured me otherwise, that I would never be able to get over his early death. However, if I could go through the summer of 1994 again, I might be able to make more sense of it.

Drew once said, 'This'll give you something to write about.' At that stage I could not even talk about his illness without crying. The idea of writing a book came to me in his homeland. I am not sure if I would ever have thought of doing so in England – perhaps the distance from London lent me a different perspective. However, I was not sure that I had enough strength to go through with it. I discussed it with Drew when I revisited his grave. The wattle tree was dying but the allamanda seemed grateful for its continued support. The only wildlife I could see was a large butterfly. It opened and closed its wings rapidly in the sun as if applauding its own beauty. 'Do it! Do it!' said the voice in my head. Then again, it had said the same thing while I swallowed Drew's pills.

Forever alert to signs and wonders, I received two jolts on the day I got back. The driver of the cab taking me home from Heathrow wore a hearing aid. I recognised him immediately. Drew and I had flagged down his taxi on Essex Road on two consecutive mornings during the second course of chemotherapy. Then, on my way to the Angel to do some shopping, I saw Drew's GP standing on the steps of his surgery, enjoying a cigarette in the afternoon air. The story was still out there after six years. I was the only character who had changed. All I had to do was tell it.

I had changed, but I knew I had not truly moved on. A can of Orangina Drew had bought was still in the fridge. The doctor, who must have signed hundreds of death certificates since Drew's, would probably not even remember him. My friends no longer talked about Drew unless I brought his name up – they had, quite rightly, got on with their lives.

So, too, had my family: Curtis, my nephew, now had a sister called Lucy; their mother was pregnant with Jack. I was touched when Linda told me that he had nearly been named Drew. Whatever, I could not love him any more than I did. I was determined to be a good uncle. They might need my help one day. I had learned how important it was to feel needed.

'Who's that?' Curtis was bouncing up and down on my bed. He pointed at the photograph of Drew.

'He's my very best friend. We used to live together in London. He's in Australia now.'

'Where my plane came from.'

'That's it.' Curtis was obsessed with trains, planes and automobiles. He had hundreds. I had bought him an inflatable Qantas jet at Cairns airport. Lucy still loved her cuddly koala. Jack had yet to be born.

'Catch me!' He launched himself into the air. My knees buckled.

'You're getting too big and I'm getting too old for this.' I dropped him back on to the mangled duvet.

'Again!'

I would have hidden the picture had my father come into the room. This knowledge added to the frustrations of yet another chaotic Christmas in Lancaster. It was ridiculous that the whole family had to maintain a conspiracy of silence to protect the feelings of the cigar-wielding patriarch. There are none so blind as those who will not see.

'Just to let you know I remembered the anniversary yesterday,' my mother had said when she rang five months earlier. 'I didn't get a chance to call.'

'Why are you whispering?'

'I don't want your father to hear. He's just gone upstairs.'

'Thank you.' And that was it.

The subject of Drew and me was an unmentionable one; my mother appeared to prefer it that way. I gave her no warning that I was going to break the silence. It took me a year to do it. This book provided the stimulus. If I was going to tell the truth then it had to be the whole truth – I had to explain what *Wrong Rooms* was going to be about.

I had grown up with guilt. It was, apparently, wrong to be gay and equally wrong to talk about it: that was why homosexuality was known as 'the love that dare not speak its name'. It did not feel wrong – when I first spent the night with that boy in Manchester nothing felt more natural – yet, even with Alex's trailblazing example, it took me years to come to terms with the fact that I was gay. I accepted it physically but not mentally. My head contradicted my heart. It was as if I was living under false pretences: I was an impostor in the changing room. Real men did not love other men. Drew taught me that they did. His love made me feel whole, removed the flaw in my character.

Alex was right: some gay men, including himself, pursued physical perfection because they felt – consciously or subconsciously – damaged inside. Their training regimes were not about health, but hedonism. However, recreational drugs undid all the hard work. 'That's the point, silly. You get wrecked. You recover. You get wrecked. You recover. That's what life's about. Pleasure and pain. Sin and repentance. Not everyone wants domestic bliss.'

The stable relationship with Drew provided me with the alibi I believed I needed. We were just as good as straights: honest, reliable, faithful. We paid more tax, used fewer services, and mostly observed the laws of the land. We were worth just as much as anyone else. The British government would not have recognised the relationship but, on a personal level, everybody else, apart from our parents, had. Furthermore, by being together, we had also achieved self-recognition.

However, no sooner had one form of guilt been banished than another took its place. Social guilt is more insidious than sexual guilt. It is much easier to change yourself than society. I did not feel guilty about keeping my promise immediately: in the first few months after Drew's death I was too numb to feel anything. The guilt crept up on me, polluted my grief, and prolonged the mourning process. Once again, my head contradicted my heart. I knew, in the eyes of the law, that I had done wrong but I felt as though I had done the right thing. I acted out of love – there was no malice aforethought – so how could I be a murderer? The law says that no one can agree to their own murder. It is illegal to assist in a suicide. There were only the two of us in that room. I had to either break my word or break the law. Drew meant everything to me. I was not going to destroy his trust or risk his love for the sake of a technicality.

And the world would have been none the wiser had I kept my mouth shut. I cannot say that I 'got away with it' because I have been living with the consequences ever since. I am already serving a life sentence. I did not care what happened to me then; in a sense, I do not care what happens to me now. However, I do care what happens to our families – and this has made a difficult task almost impossible. The truth matters. Drew's story is by no means unique but I believe it should be told.

*

On 1 June 2001 Uncle Mark attended Curtis's sixth birthday party. Screaming kids, piles of presents, lots of ice-cream: we had such a good time. My sister was exhausted. Baby Jack, however, kindly slept through the carnival mayhem. It must be wonderful to have made new life out of your love, to see yourselves in your children, to know that, after you have gone, you will live on through them. Meanwhile, though, bringing them up was hell.

'I won't mind if one of them turns out to be gay,' Linda once told me. 'I just want them to be happy.' I remembered her words the next morning as I walked down Piggy Lane with my father. He was bound to be disappointed: I was the end of the Sanderson line. We stopped in the Millennium Garden that had once been the orchard of a house on Cannon Hill. The meadow grass needed mowing but the work experience lads had done a good job. The mica in a stone bench glinted in the sun. I needed to sit down. My father sat down painfully beside me.

'Before I tell you what *Wrong Rooms* is about I need to tell you something else. It will probably upset you, and I'm sorry for that, but it's better that you hear it from me than anyone else.' My father looked at me hard. He was an old man racked with arthritis yet I was still afraid of him.

'Do it! Do it!' said the voice.

'I'm gay. Always have been and always will be.'

'Yes. I know.' There was no surprise, no anger.

'Well, why didn't you say anything?'

'I thought it was for you to tell me.'

'Mum asked me not to.' Now he was surprised. 'She said it would kill you.'

'Oh.'

'Did you guess that Drew and I were lovers?'

'You seemed very close. It was obvious that his death knocked you sideways.'

'That's one way of putting it.'

'Keep going! Keep going!' said the voice.

'Do you remember telling Mum, years and years ago, that she had to put you out of your misery if an accident left you in a persistent coma?'

'I've no wish to be a vegetable if that's what you mean. I couldn't bear to lie there day after day. Waiting to die is not living.'

'Well, Drew asked me to do the same. I suffocated him.'

'I take it that's what he wanted.'

'In the end it was. I didn't do it against his will!' Did he really think I was capable of murder?

'Have you spoken to a lawyer?'

'My agent dragged me there himself. I don't care what happens to me. If the worst came to the worst I could say I'd made it all up – there's no proof either way – but the whole point of the book is to tell the truth. I can't keep it to myself any more. I'll go mad. In fact I think I've been out of my mind ever since his death. I won't be able to come to terms with it until I've made a complete confession.'

'What about his parents? Have you told them? How will they take the news?'

'I don't know. I've decided to tell them as soon as I've finished the book. If I finish it. I'm not sure that I'll be able to go through with it.'

A boxer puppy bounded up and started sniffing our feet. 'Brontë! Brontë!' Her young owner and three of his mates emerged from the bushes. 'She won't bite, she's just nosy.' The dog made friends with my father wetly. The boys tramped on. I was old enough to be their father. No doubt they would give their real fathers an equally hard time. That was what sons did.

I was surprised at the restraint of my father's reaction. My relief was mixed with joy and regret. I wished I had told him sooner. I had underestimated him. I felt closer to him already. Chat did change things sometimes. We continued to talk as we made our way home. I stressed that I was apologising for any trouble I might cause, not for the fact that I was gay. 'I have to be true to myself. You always told me it doesn't matter what other people think – and I do know what you think about raving homosexuals.'

'You're still my son, though. I'll always be here for you.'

My mother looked relieved when I told her that the secret was out. Her voice on the telephone had filled with dread at the prospect of a book about Drew's illness and death. The years of feigning ignorance were over. They must have been quite a strain. I was beginning to understand that her first allegiance had always been to my father in the same way that mine had eventually been to Drew. I left it to my father to explain exactly how Drew had died. It was her turn to be the last to know now.

In the early hours of 16 July I followed the usual routine. I lit the scented candle, sat on Drew's bed and sobbed my heart out. I had completed Chapter 3 the day before. The worst times loomed ahead.

Happy endings only happen in books but this one cannot end happily. Drew can never come back. However, this book's very existence is a kind of happy ending. The fact that I am still here, writing at the desk in this room, astonishes me. Cancer nearly destroyed the two of us. Perhaps miracles do take place after all. Whatever happens now, our story will outlive us.

Each night, before I turn out the light, I kiss Drew's pillow. I still talk to him. His crucifix is still round my neck. Drew never owned a mobile phone or had an e-mail address. He never turned on a widescreen television to laugh at *Big Brother* or tuned in to hear Fat Boy Slim – right here, right now – on a digital radio station. It is almost eight years since he died and yet in some ways it seems like seconds.

While I knew how much I loved Drew, writing *Wrong Rooms* has revealed how much he loved me. His room is not a crime scene: what happened in it was a love scene. The pain in my left shoulder has lessened since the osteopath insisted I buy a new pillow. I threw the old one away. The migraines are under control too. Even the nightmare has faded. The figure at the end of the bed turned out to be me: an ordinary man needing to love and be loved. You cannot deny who you are for ever. On the other hand, the person who began this book no longer exists. The completion of it has been an ordeal. I lost Drew all over again but, in the process, set myself free. I have finally learned that letting go is a sign of strength, not weakness.

Is it possible to love someone too much? Did I do the right thing? No doubt the world will tell me. I am, however, certain of this: I would do anything to spend ten seconds more in his arms.

Epilogue

A ileen told Jack to turn off the television. Blackness, like the curtains in a cinema, swept across the widescreen from both sides.

'Did Drew ever mention a promise?'

'No.' His mother shook her head. I was not surprised: he would not have wanted to upset them. They would probably have tried to talk him out of it anyway. I would have to spell it out.

'After his first course of chemo he made me promise that I'd help him die if he decided he couldn't take any more.' I breathed in deeply.

'I thought someone might have tampered with his morphine pump,' said Aileen. 'The end came sooner than we expected.'

So they had suspected something. At least the news would not come as a total shock.

'I'm convinced Drew would have died on the sixteenth regardless. I thought I'd left it too late but he was determined to fight for as long as he could. I didn't touch the morphine pump: I was afraid it would take too long.'

'The dosage was carefully calibrated,' said Jack. 'They would have noticed anything amiss.'

'I hated the nameplate on it,' said Aileen. The pump had been paid for by the parents of a little girl. A plastic plaque marked their generosity – and reminded other patients that the device would outlast them too. 'It was morbid.'

'I still feel sick if my cab goes past the Middlesex. I avoid Mortimer Street whenever I can.' For a moment there was silence.

'So how did you do it?' said Aileen. I forced myself to meet her gaze.

'Well, he could no longer swallow so . . . I used a pillow.'

'He was unconscious. How can you be sure that's what he wanted?'

'Believe me, he wasn't unconscious. It scares me now that he was conscious more than we thought. He couldn't speak that night but I made absolutely sure he knew what I was about to do. He gave me the go-ahead. There was no doubt about it. I didn't want to do it. Right up to the last minute I hoped he would change his mind. I didn't want to do it, but I did. I loved him so much.'

All three of us were close to tears. Ming-Ming, sensing the tension, miaowed. For once she was ignored. I remained silent. There was nothing else to say.

Eventually Aileen said, 'I understand why you did it but at

the moment I don't like how you did it. The thought of a pillow over little Drew's face . . .' Her voice quavered. 'Asphyxiation is very painful.'

'He was in a hell of a lot of pain already,' said Jack.

As I had lain awake in the small hours, night after night, I had envisaged various scenarios: screams, violence, instant ejection. None of them was played out. In the event the one thing that I had not thought of happened: his parents heard me out calmly and quietly. I offered to leave, to let them consider the news in private, but they said there was no need. Aileen shared out the remains of the Yellowglen. I was grateful for the alcohol. I was shaking. They asked me about the legal repercussions of the book. I was amazed at their concern for my welfare. I should not have been: after all, these kind people had brought up Drew.

We went to a nearby restaurant as planned. The whole meal had an air of surreal normality. Overcome with exhaustion and relief, I could hardly eat. Back at the house, before I left, Aileen took a photograph of me and Jack. I was part of the family at last.

There was no one on Ghost Beach. I had the island to myself. Lizard Island, where I was staying, lay across the warm, clear waters of the Blue Lagoon. I had climbed up to Cook's Look, its highest point, the day before. The Captain, whose ships were trapped, had been searching for a way out of the Great Barrier Reef and, eventually, had found it. London, according to the bronze dial at the summit, was 14,900 kilometres away.

The flight from Cairns had taken fifty-five minutes. A journey that, in one sense, had started in September 1992 had finally reached its end. Drew would have loved it here. Green hills, turquoise sea, yellow sun. Total tranquillity. An eagle flew so low over my head I could hear the air rushing beneath its wings. Without Drew I would not have discovered this idyllic spot. Now I was without him again. He was never coming back. I would never stop loving him. He had fought for his life for as long as he could. The best way I could celebrate his memory was by making the most of my own.

The dying waves hissed about my feet. Once upon a time, the fact that Drew was not here, building a castle on the beach, would have filled me with rage: not any more. Drew had changed my life and now the remembrance of his love had given me the courage to change my life again.

A week later I returned to Cairns. I half expected to be met by two mirror-shaded policemen at the airport. A part of me will always feel guilty. His parents might have had second thoughts, become enraged as the news had sunk in, demanded retribution. As soon as I smelled the lily-of-the-valley perfume I knew they had not. Aileen liked her present. We chatted for a couple of hours – about Drew, Jack's successful eye operation and this book – but not about what happened on 16 July. The future was what counted now.

A taxi sounded its horn. It was time to go home. I hugged his mother and shook hands with his father.

'You're doing a good thing,' he said.